Yoga
For a Healthy Body

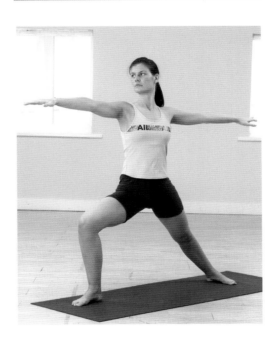

HEALTH LEARNING CENTER
Northwestern Memorial Hospital
Galter 3-304
Chicago, IL

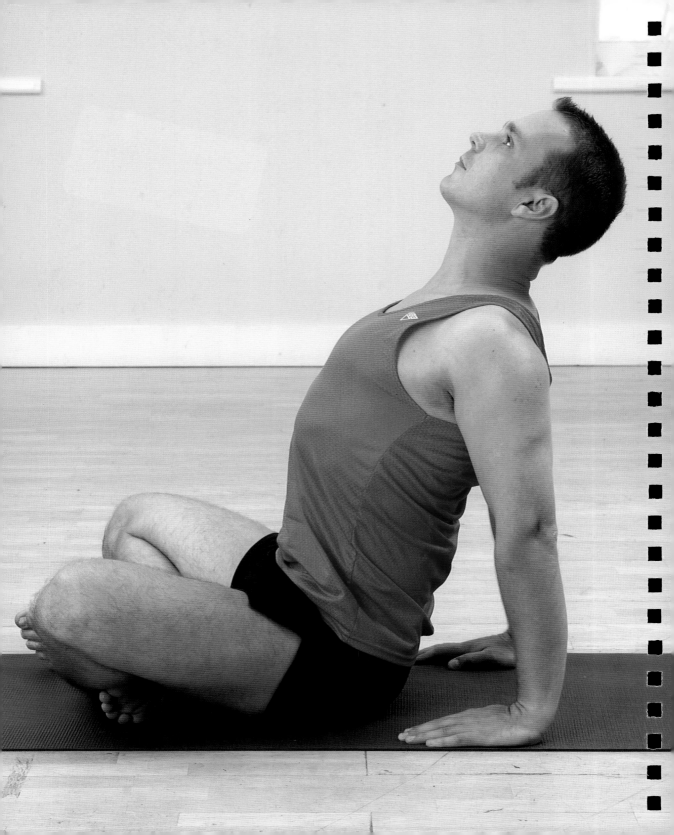

Yoga
For a Healthy Body

A STEP-BY-STEP GUIDE

COMBINE EXERCISE AND MEDITATION

20-MINUTE WORKOUTS

Imelda Maguire

Main Street
A division of Sterling Publishing Co., Inc.
New York

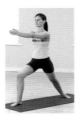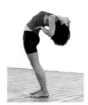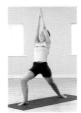

Library of Congress Cataloging-in-Publication Data Available

10 9 8 7 6 5 4 3 2 1

Published by Main Street a division of Sterling Publishing Co., Inc.
387 Park Avenue South, New York, NY 10016
© 2005 by PRC Publishing
An imprint of **Chrysalis** Books Group plc

Distributed in Canada by Sterling Publishing
c/o Canadian Manda Group, 165 Dufferin Street
Toronto, Ontario, Canada M6K 3H6

Printed in China

1 4027 1966 3

The exercise programs described in this book are based on well-established
practices proven to be effective for over-all health and fitness, but they are
not a substitute for personalized advice from a qualified practitioner. Always
consult with a qualified health care professional in matters relating to your
health before beginning this or any exercise program. This is especially
important if you are pregnant or nursing, if you are elderly, or if you have
any chronic or recurring medical condition. As with any exercise program,
if at any point during your workout you begin to feel faint, dizzy, or have
physical discomfort, you should stop immediately and consult a physician.

The purpose of this book is to educate and is sold with the
understanding that the author and the publisher shall have neither liability
nor responsibility for any injury caused or alleged to be caused directly
or indirectly by the information contained in this book.

Contents

Introduction

Yoga is an ancient system of exercise from India. Yoga comes from the Indian word *yuj*, which means to bind together, to join, or to unite. It is the union of the mind, body, and spirit—a holistic approach to your physical and mental well-being. It is a system of exercise that combines stretching and breathing with a relaxed awareness, resulting in a beautiful, toned body, glowing complexion, and a positive attitude toward life.

The practice of yoga teaches us to take responsibility for ourselves, for our physical and mental well-being, teaching us to respond to the needs of the moment with sensitivity, grace, and ease.

Everyone can practice yoga. It is for everybody. We all have a body that can be trained in some manner. The thoughtful practice of yoga promotes a mental and physical flexibility that students find beneficial in all areas of life, unlimited by concerns of ageing, sex, or strength. All you need is comfortable clothing, a mat to practice on and the firm determination to do something about your life. Yoga's gifts are accessible to everybody and it can help to develop balance, flexibility, vitality, and strength. Yoga also reduces stress, increases awareness, and calms the mind.

The aim of this book is to introduce you to a series of movements and breathing techniques which will enable you to calm down, tone up, and feel great.

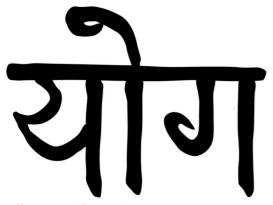

Yoga means unification—the union of the body and the mind.

Hatha yoga

The yoga in this book is known as Hatha yoga. This is an activity that is health-giving in the fullest sense of the word. It is very much a holistic approach to health, which considers diet and nutrition. It is a mindful approach to exercise, rather than a mindless one. It is an approach to life that will pervade a person's whole way of being.

Hatha yoga is the union of opposites. "Ha" translates as sun, "tha" as moon and literally means the union of the sun and moon. The sun is symbolized by the in breath. It represents expansion, movement, the body, and the positive. The moon is symbolized by the out breath. It represents contraction, stillness, the mind, and the negative. The union of the in breath and out breath is the harmony realized when the body and mind are balanced and at ease. It is also the union of all the different aspects of ourselves. The union of ourselves with the universe.

The movements called postures (asanas), are designed to work each muscle, joint, and ligament in the body, stimulating the circulation and nourishing each cell for optimum health and vitality. The breathing rhythms of yoga enable us to access the life force within us, creating vigor, vitality, and a tranquil mind.

Hatha yoga should be easy and taken gently. Over-exertion works against the practitioner. Hatha yoga should be practiced slowly, mindfully, and with a free-flowing breath and a quiet mind. The practice should leave the practitioner feeling full of energy, not tired out, as you would after intense athletic activity. Pain has its use, but only as an indicator of getting things wrong, of missing the way, and it helps lead us back to the path of harmony.

Hatha yoga is a purificatory process of cleansing and toning the body and mind. It is practiced as the first step to all yogic disciplines. Its aim is to cease the endless chitter chatter of the mind so the light of your true self will shine.

The eight fold path to liberation

Over two thousand years ago, Patanjali, a great Indian sage, set out the principles and practices of yoga which he called the "eight fold path to liberation." This is known as Raja yoga, the royal path, or the path to liberation. A brief outline of the eight paths follows:

1. **Yama:** Abstinences. Not doing any physical, verbal or mental violence against yourself or others. Moral restraint and control in thought, word, and deed. Social conduct and examples we set for the harmonious functioning of society.

2. **Niyama:** Observances. Things to do, such as personal cleanliness or studying. Having purity in thought and deed, contentment, surrender of the ego, and directing your life toward truth.

3. **Asanas:** Postures. Steady poses for a healthy, functioning body that rids ourselves of physical and psychosomatic tensions, so we may experience stillness; within and without.

4. **Pranayama:** Expansion of the breath. Control of vital energy.

5. **Pratyahara:** Withdrawal of the senses. Taking us away from the body image. Looking within. Being centered and calm.

6. **Dharana:** Concentration of the mind. Being focused. The ability to control our energy and harness our imagination.

7. **Dhyana:** Meditation. Finding peace in everything you do. The mind is still and no longer wanders. Being at peace.

8. **Samadhi:** Enlightenment. Self-realization. Being at one with the universe. Enjoying a connection to all life.

This eight fold path, known as the sutras of Patanjali, may be likened to tools or aids, steps along the way, which enable us to understand and develop ourselves. They help us to accept gladly all the adverse circumstances that arise, regarding them as opportunities to learn and develop, rather than lamenting the situation in which we find ourselves.

Physical health is not seen as an aim in itself, but as a means to developing self-awareness. In yoga it is not how well you perform the postures, rather the intensity and direction of your efforts. Yoga is finding peace in whatever you do, be it washing the dishes, driving a car, mowing the lawn, going to work, or looking at the stars. Do not think about what you could be doing. Rather, find peace in what you are doing. As long as you find yourself doing that particular thing, you might as well enjoy it. Doing this you find peace within yourself.

The aim of Patanjali's yoga sutras is to arrive at a state of bliss and joy called samadhi. This is achieved by the steady persistence and practice of control over our physical and mental agitations, allowing us to connect to the fine forces that lie beneath the flesh, and thereby gain independence and freedom from the

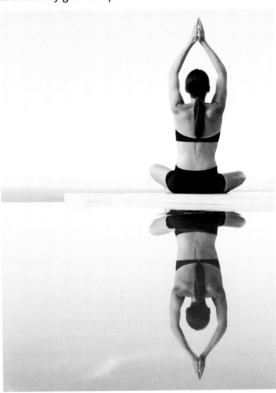

body image. The practice of the sutras provides a firm foundation for success. A state in which the body and mind remain in harmony under all circumstances. If you choose to practice the postures without taking on board the eight steps you are not practicing yoga, merely indulging in yogic exercises.

Yama

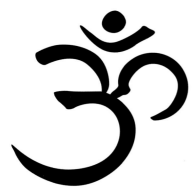

Om written in Sanskrit

Yama is abstinence or restraint. The most important aspects of the yoga steps are the practice of yama (non-violence) and niyama (self improvement).

Negative feelings, such as violence, are damaging to our life, whether we act upon them ourselves or cause or condone them in others. When we are firmly established in non-violence, all beings around us cease to feel hostility. Incorporating yama into our yoga practice means no pain. That pain only has its use as an indicator of missing the way and guides us back to the path of harmony.

Patanjali stated that in order to get rid of painful thoughts, disturbing feelings, and morbid habits of mind, we must dwell constantly on the opposite. The body soon begins to respond to happy, buoyant thoughts, encouraging a simple and positive approach to life, enabling us to experience sameness toward our friends as well as our enemies.

To those who are good be good, to those who are bad be also good, that way goodness is achieved. Instead of wasting your energy on deliberately feeding negative emotions and situations, direct that energy into positive, peaceful actions and thoughts.

Yama literally translates as "restraint." By tradition there are five restraints: abstention from violence, falsehood, stealing, sensuality, and greed. These are expressed positively as gentleness, truthfulness, honesty, temperance, and generosity. How do we apply them? By bringing our yoga principles into our home and workplace, applying them to our family, friends, and colleagues. This means directly setting out to make life as happy and harmonious as possible, no matter how difficult this is to achieve. By setting an example, cooperating, leading when necessary, and not losing your temper! It also means loving discipline to children, complete honesty between partners, and understanding and fulfillment of each other's needs. These constitute yama, the firm determination to do something about your life.

Niyama

With niyama there are five observances in the conduct toward oneself. They are cleanliness, contentment, examination of the senses, austerity, and devotion to an ideal.

Cleanliness applies to thought, deed, body, and mind. It is important to maintain a high standard of personal hygiene. This includes elimination of residues and impurities from the internal organs, the digestive tract, the lungs, and the nasal passages. Niyama focuses on personal development with a corresponding increase in humility and love.

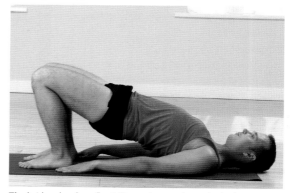

The bridge develops flexibility and strengthens the back.

Asanas

Asanas are postures, the third step of Patanjali's yoga sutras. They are used for balance, sound health, and to tone up every part of the body. The asanas remove physical and psychosomatic tensions, so we can sit in comfort, concentrate, and meditate without bodily distraction. The endocrine system (certain ductless glands, thyroid, and thymus) are stimulated, which helps maintain good health and a feeling of well-being. Energy is directed away from the body image and channeled to positive ends. The body is a temple of the self and the practice of the postures will keep it healthy and full of vitality. The effects of the postures can be summed up as, "That which you nourish grows, that which you neglect dies."

Pranayama

Pranayama is the expansion of the breath. There is no need for complicated, repetitive routines. Unhurried living results in unhurried breathing. By listening to the breath, becoming aware of the movement of the breath, without effort, we learn to recognize the changes and nuances in our breath. We gain an understanding of how our breathing rhythm is affected by our emotions. Pranayama is an ideal method for producing calmness and tranquility. When your breath is calm, your mind is calm.

Pratyahara

Sense withdrawal, pratyahara, is the fifth step on the path. It is a detachment from physical, emotional, and mental activity; the ability to hold a posture with grace and ease without the need to fidget or change your position. The mind is free to concentrate without bodily interference. We learn to harness our latent energies, direct, and control them. We are unconcerned about our image, we seek no distractions to our inner and outer equilibrium.

Dharana

Concentration, or dharana, is the cornerstone of mind control. Concentration helps us to focus on the matter

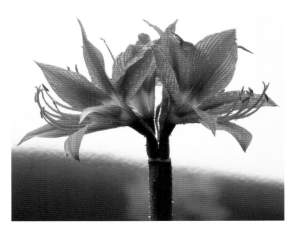
A flower can focus the mind.

in hand, conserving energy, and calming the emotions. Powers of observation and memory are improved and greater control over one's thoughts and actions are rapidly developed. Concentration brings about peace of mind. When the mind is focused on one thing at a time it cannot be fragmented or harassed. Concentration is impeded by tension and tension increases pain. So release the tension! You can concentrate on anything to focus your wandering mind, such as the sound of the wind or birdsong. You can gaze at a candle, shell, or flower, or you can just listen to your breathing and allow the movement of your breath to calm, relax, and guide you.

Dhyana

Dhyana is meditation. Finding peace in everything you do is the aim of meditation practice as well as finding our core, our center, understanding our inner nature, and developing wisdom.

Samadhi

Samadhi is contemplation. The achievement of complete harmony and control within and without. The body, mind, and spirit (breath) are one unified whole. The soul enjoys silence and peace by simply contemplating the truth.

Schools of Yoga

There are many schools and disciplines in yoga. If we liken them to pearls on a necklace, hatha yoga is the thread that binds them. Hatha yoga is the basis for all yoga practices. We start with hatha yoga and develop along the yogic path best suited to our needs and temperament. Only by choosing the path most relevant to our daily life can we expect to be successful. Hatha yoga is often described as the yoga of the breath or the science of the breath. We learn to resonate with our breath and be guided by it. If you practice the postures without following the breath, once again there is no yoga, merely athletics. The practice of the postures eliminates obstacles, which our body might put in the way of self-realization.

Bhakti yoga

Bhakti yoga is the yoga of love and devotion. The love of the bhakti yogi must be all-embracing and unquestioning, with no expectation of return of this love, similar to that of a mother's love for their child. Before embarking on this path, the bhakti yogi must

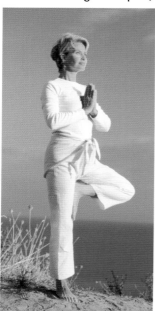

look in his/her heart to see if they have this type of selflessness. The bhakti yogi must give exactly the same quality of love to their family, friends, neighbors, and enemies. They must look to find the goodness in all things.

The yogi strives to find goodness to eclipse the bad aspects. In this way the yogi finds similarities with all things and recognizes their place in the universe. Fire burns, but also warms.

You can drown in water but it is also thirst quenching. There is a negative and positive aspect to all creation, we try to seek out the good and encourage it.

The bhakti yogi trains herself/himself to approach good and evil with equanimity, knowing that the power of love and good will enhance everything. The bhakti yogi sees God (the universal spirit) in everything, and expands this goodness to the universe. It is often referred to as the yoga for women devoted to the home and family, with the selfless love for a person or an ideal.

Bhakti yoga is the path of divine love in which the emotions are purified by the sublimation of desires and lusts into a perfect joy. This is accomplished through devotion and adoration of a teacher or guru or some being that sets a divine example for concentrated effort. The bhakti yogi must be careful not to fritter away divine energies on ceremony or pomp, but should concentrate on all that is pure, selfless , harmless, and loving.

Jnana yoga

Jnana yoga is the yoga of knowledge and discrimination. It is an inward-looking philosophy based on the belief that innate, true wisdom is intuitive knowledge. The jnana yogi, in an effort to understand man and his place in the universe, must first fully understand him/herself, and gain complete control over his/her body and mind. He or she renounces all superficial mental and physical activities, the better to concentrate all energies on gaining insight. In this respect, this is not the type of yoga for the person who loves to socialize, as this wastes much effort and energy.

At each turn the jnani yogi must decide between right and wrong, importance and trivia, virtue and vice. They must have the moral strength not only to believe in their judgment but also to act on it. They must seek to find their own depths, before turning attention to the universe.

The jnani yogi practices penance or self-sacrifice in order to master their appetites and not be ruled by them. Jnana is the giving of self, one's duty to society.

This is practiced in the help given to parents, family, and friends in acknowledgment of all they have done; accepting the debt for all that has been received. Teaching yoga is an example of jnana yoga.

The duties the yogi performs are not only for the benefit of mankind, but also toward their own spiritual progress. The idea is not to be arrogant, never saying I told you so, not to waste time on gossip or unnecessary activities. Their search is for the ultimate and all other mental activities must cease. The search is for peace and tranquility. Knowing others is wisdom, knowing yourself is enlightenment.

Finally, it must be emphasized that although the jnana yogi tend to cut themselves off from a lot of social activities, they are not hermits and do not reject society. Rather, from their constant meditation and search for truth, they set an example to all. It is often said that if society as a whole could call upon the jnana yogi, the whole of society would benefit from their peaceful and calm counseling. They do not quarrel, so no one quarrels with them.

Karma yoga

Karma yoga is the yoga of action. The word karma is connected to the sanskrit word *kri*, which is all about the creation of work coupled with action and spiritual ritual. Every work in life, however humble, can become an act of creation or a means of salvation, as we reconcile the finite with the infinite. Karma yoga is perfect action with a loving attitude.

Actions speak louder than words and we work to lose our karma, which is our preconditioned response to life. Karma consists of samskars or memories, which are manifested as skills, habits, and tendencies. Karma is not about what you have done in the past, it's about responding to the needs of the moment, things that are in the here and now—how you act, once you are awake and aware.

The wheel of karma revolves and although we must work with love in our hearts, the work is not for a reward, but in the knowledge that whatever we think we will become.

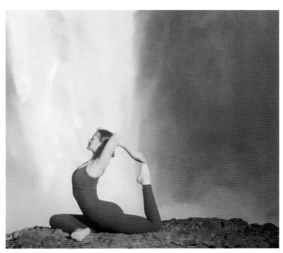

The yogi is free of karma when only the self in its pure form remains. Karma yoga is the transcending of pain from our past lives and recent actions.

Nurses, doctors, and teachers are an example of karma yoga in action. As the maitri Upanis once described, "Samara, the transmigration of life, takes place in one's own mind. Let us therefore keep the mind pure, for what a man thinks he becomes: this is a mystery of eternity."

Raja yoga

Known as the royal path or the yoga of the will, raja yoga embraces all the yogic paths. It is the spiritual way taught in all the great philosophies of the world. The pathway leads inward toward your own inner god-like self.

Raja yoga is the combination of all the yoga paths which intermingle and overlap. Practicing hatha yoga we eliminate the obstacles our body might put in the way of self-realization. In karma yoga, we purify our actions and achieve detachment from the results. In bhakti yoga, we intensify the power of love. With jnana yoga we find that knowledge and freedom are within us.

Practicing hatha, we may become obsessed with the competitive spirit, needing the detachment of karma yoga, to refrain from performing postures too difficult for an ill-prepared body. For karma yoga, we need the all-embracing love of bhakti yoga in order to perform our actions well. Jnana yoga provides the knowledge and discrimination between worthy and unworthy actions and aims.

The bhakti yogi must practice sufficient hatha to keep their body fit, and karma yoga to provide the detachment which ensures that they will not be downcast when the object of their devotion does not reciprocate their love.

The jnana yogi cannot be effective without the compassion of bhakti, to ensure humility, karma, to ensure tenacity of purpose, and hatha, to control the mind and body.

Laya yoga, merges the mind with the self through one-pointed concentration on sounds and ideas. Not only is a still mind called for, but a fervent focus of the imagination upon the divine as well.

Laya yoga includes japa, a rhythmic repetition of mantras and other spiritual formulae. This is used to fire and transform the imagination and to rid the mind of gloom, fear, and anxieties by concentrating on its opposites, that is, optimism and joy.

Yantra is also included and this is the visual aid to understanding through symbolic form—designs composed of interlaced triangles, figures, and symbols as aids to meditation and ritual. Circular designs are known as mandalas, and are associated with peace and love.

Mantra is the repetition of specific words and sounds (like a cat purring) to produce good health and power which can be used for healing purposes.

The true spirit of laya yoga is one in which we renounce all things that bind and blind our true self—not out of fear, but out of a deep longing to regain true freedom.

Tantric yoga is about the ability to raise kundalini energy. The symbolism is of a sleeping snake coiled three and a half times and lying at the base of the spine. Through various techniques, the snake is woken and rises up the length of the spine, opening and stimulating energy centers, called chakras, along the way. The aim is to unite your male and female energies, raise your consciousness, and enjoy a state of joy and bliss.

Traditional hatha yoga is the most popular form of yoga practiced today. You will find hatha yoga classes taught in schools, gyms, and leisure centers.

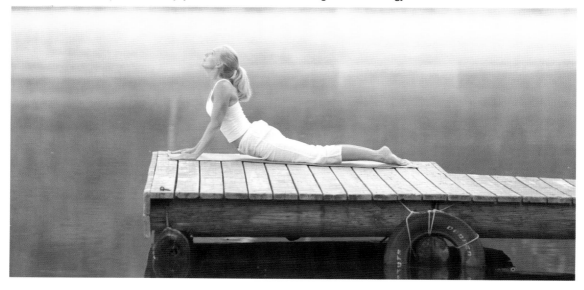

Twenty-first Century Yoga

Astanga vinyasa yoga

Astanga vinyasa yoga is growing in popularity as it incorporates all the features that are most attractive within an aerobic workout. Yet it also gives the inner fulfillment that the ancient practice of yoga is known for. Dance-like, dynamic, flowing movements that lend freedom of expression to the body are part of a choreographed sequential form.

Vinyasa yoga stands apart from most other forms of yoga practice because its main features are a constant physical activity and a heightened energy level. By combining the control and discipline of classical hatha yoga, with the excitement of dance, aerobic exercise, and body sculpting, vinyasa yoga gives the body a balanced development of physical strength. It is also used as a therapy, because continual and regular practice helps free the muscular system, allowing the skeleton to regain its correct alignment, encouraging good posture and excellent body tone. Vinyasa yoga is the most physically involved form, serving as a path to health, flexibility, balance, and control, with great emphasis on concentration and attitude. Vinyasa yoga is divided into six different series, each one working and concentrating on a different aspect of the individual.

The warrior creates flexibility in the hips.

Iyengar yoga

Iyengar yoga is a system of yoga devised by Mr. B.K.S. Iyengar. It is hatha yoga in all its glory, with the accompaniment of aids, blocks, and bands to help the student into position. Once a student becomes qualified to teach Iyengar yoga, they can teach no other style, as this is a purist style with schools worldwide. It is dynamic and progressive.

Other forms of yoga

Sivananda yoga has centers all around the world. It is deep, spiritual, and practical. Bikram yoga is practiced in a hot room and is a specific, choreographed sequence of dynamic postures. Anusura yoga is John Friend's unique style of yoga, which works on precise alignment and spiritual values. John teaches that everything in the world is an expression of the divine—your smile, your dog, even your car. The aim is to unite with the divine and express this union through mind, body, and spirit. It is big and fun and quintessentially American. Power yoga is an offshoot of astanga yoga. The poses are powerful and dynamic. Unlike astanga yoga, the flowing sequence is not the same every time.

In traditional yoga practice there is often a reference to God. You may prefer to relate to this word as creator, cosmos, universe, or nature.

In thinking of God, we are connecting to that which is divine. In yogic philosophy the divine is unadulterated freedom. The aim is to connect with the divine in all things and to see the beauty in all things. The spirit is that which is inherent in all living things—that is, the breath. The spirit can be refined, polished, and perfected during the whole of one's life.

"Let your spirit be your true shield."
Morihei Ueshiba

Yoga Basics

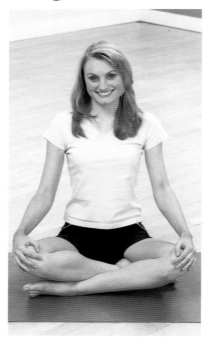

Sit cross-legged for breathing exercises.

terrible way to live. Find a mental picture that gives you pleasure and immediately switch your scary thought to a pleasurable thought. Plant your own garden and cultivate your soul, instead of waiting for someone to bring you flowers. As you progress, you will find the practice of yoga begins to take you away from the body image or how fat or thin you are. Your attitude changes to "How do I feel?" not "How do I look?"

As we become accustomed to feeling toned from the inside, we consciously choose foods and a lifestyle that promote this feeling of well-being. Yoga produces a feeling of lightness and vitality. This is experienced in the mind also. As we learn to let go and release physical and psychosomatic tension, we recognize that our thoughts and attitudes make our life what it is. As the Buddha said:

We are our thoughts.
Everything we do arises with our thoughts.
With our thoughts
We make our world.

Mental attitude

Approach your yoga practice with a smile. You know you are going to feel better the moment you start. Remember it's fun and makes you feel good.

The practice of yama and niyama (physical and mental conduct) enable us to approach our practice with grace and equanimity. Think of practicing as a time to pamper yourself physically and mentally.

Be gentle, kind, and patient with yourself as you learn new ways of thinking and responding.

Praise yourself. Criticism breaks down our inner spirit, praise builds it up. Tell yourself how well you are doing. Accept yourself as you are. Refuse to criticize yourself. Everybody changes. When you criticize yourself, your changes are negative, when you approve of yourself, your changes are positive.

Do not terrorize yourself with your thoughts, it is a

So if you want to change yourself and your world, change your thoughts. Think of light. Think of love.

Breathing

It has been said that a man counts his life in years, a yogi in the amount of breaths he takes. The breath, postures, and emotions are linked. Listen to your breathing. Is it smooth, deep, and rhythmic? Or is it short, shallow, and ragged? Deep, rhythmic breathing produces vitality and the ability to think clearly. Short, shallow breathing brings tension, anxiety, and irritability. With practice we learn to observe our breath and the changes that occur in breathing; whether we are active or still, tense or relaxed, happy or sad.

Recognizing these feelings, emotions, and tensions, we learn to consciously relax and let go of negative emotions and embrace a positive approach to life. The breath, its rhythm and depth, is the focus of our attention. No complicated routines are necessary for this. Listening to your breath automatically detaches you from the worries and the anxieties of your mind. When your breath is calm, your mind is calm also. When your mind is calm, your body responds by moving gracefully.

When we first start listening to the breath, we become aware of the sound and quality of our breath. Then we become aware of the rise of the chest as we inhale, the fall of our chest as we exhale. We can imagine our lungs to be like a pair of balloons; when we breathe in the lungs expand and fill, when we breathe out, the lungs contract and empty.

Our breathing becomes quieter as we realize that listening to the breath is in reality an internal listening. It's not about how quiet or noisy our breath is. It's more a connection made to how you really are at this moment in time. Not how you look or how you feel.

Sometimes, when looking introspectively, we experience feelings of sadness, frustration, and anger. This is normal. The trick is not to hang on to these feelings. Breathe these negative anxieties out.

> "Pain of the past-future fear
> Fade away and disappear
> Into the moment of now and here
> Love is the essence within
> She heals all the wounds of the soul there have been
> She puts you together and tears you apart
> To come closer to the source and sacred heart
> Bless all the tears and sorrow
> For they are keys to a new tomorrow
> Surrender to the highest source inside
> And all shadows will dissolve into the night."
>
> Kailish

Concentration on the breath is called pranayama or breath expansion. "Pran" translates as energy/life

force, "ayam" as expansion. It is the life-giving energy that is inherent in all things, common to all life. It is universal. We absorb prana from food, water, sunlight, our parents, contact with the earth, but mainly from the air we breathe. It is accumulated through serenity but dissipated through anger and anxiety. Children have an abundance of prana.

Prana is to the Indians what *chi* is to the Chinese, and *ki* to the Koreans and Japanese. It is vital, intrinsic energy that can be harnessed and channeled to increase good health and vitality. Ancient healing traditions such as acupressure, acupuncture, and ayuveda recognize this energy, the imbalances that can occur and how to correct any illnesses caused by the imbalance.

Breathing deeply increases our life force. We can increase the capacity of our lungs just by becoming aware of our breathing. Exhaling deeply increases the release of toxins and carbons from the body. It follows that the greater your out breath, the more room you have in the lungs for clear, fresh oxygen to refresh and revitalize you.

Your breath must never be forced or strained. The breath guides us into the poses, enables us to hold the postures with ease, and guides us out of the poses and into serenity. Yogic breathing is a wonderful complement to athletic activity, increasing vitality and aiding focus and concentration. The aim of the practice of pranayama is to rid the body of toxins, to purify the mind and produce a relaxed body and a clear mind.

> "Now and again, it is necessary to seclude yourself amongst deep mountains and hidden valleys to restore your link to the source of life. Breathe in and let yourself soar to the ends of the universe; breathe out and bring the cosmos back inside. Next, breathe up all the fecundity and vibrancy of the earth. Finally, blend the breath of heaven and the breath of earth with that of your own, becoming the breath of life itself."
>
> Morihei Ueshiba

Breathing Techniques

Alternate nostril breathing (anuloma viloma)

Known as the crown of hatha yoga practices, alternate nostril breathing balances the life forces of the sun and moon, inhalation and exhalation, the right and left. It strengthens and cleanses the respiratory system, harmonizes the breath, and calms the mind.

Holding a finger or thumb over the other nostril, we inhale through the right nostril for a count of four, hold the breath to a count of four, breathe out through the left nostril for a count of sixteen. Breathe in through the left nostril for a count of four, hold the breath for a count of four, breathe out through the right nostril for a count of sixteen. Then repeat at least four times.

Beginners often begin with a ratio of breathing in for a count of two, holding for a count of two, breathing out for a count of eight. Practice and progress go hand in hand.

Ujjayi breathing (warrior breath/fire breath)

This is dynamic, rhythmic breathing; inhalation to a count of four, exhalation to a count of four. There is no pause between the breath. The rhythm is smooth and flowing, it heats up the body from the inside to the outside. It rids the body of poisons, the mind of anxieties, and warms us in preparation for the dynamic postures. Ujjayi breathing is an integral part of Astanga vinyasa yoga.

Bellows breath

The "bellows breath" fans the gastric fires. It aids digestion and the elimination of waste products from the body. It gives a feeling of lightness, both mentally and physically. After inhalation, the breath is expelled forcibly through the nostrils, the breathing is quick and rhythmic. Practice for ten breaths, rest, and then repeat three times.

Bee's breath.

The "bee's breath" produces vitality and a feeling of lightness. The tip of the tongue is placed at the top of the mouth behind the teeth. The mouth is closed. After inhalation through the nostrils, exhale through the nostrils. Make the "mmmmmmm" sound. You will feel yourself vibrating like a bee, stimulating your life force and aiding your concentration and meditation.

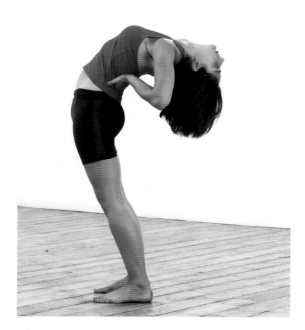

"All the principles of heaven and earth are living inside you. Life itself is the truth, and this will never change. Everything in heaven and earth breathes. Breath is the thread that ties creation together. When the myriad variations in the universal breath can be sensed, the individual techniques of the Art of Peace are born."

Morihei Ueshiba

Movement

The movements in yoga are called asanas or postures, which should be smooth-flowing, graceful, and dance-like. There is no stress or strain, pain only having its use as an indicator of missing the way, to lead us back to the path of harmony. We have to learn to listen to what our body is trying to tell us, taking responsibility for ourselves thereby avoiding the dangers of strain or injury. We must avoid competition, going only as far as we comfortably can in a pose, recognizing that over-exertion works against us and is a common mistake.

"If we wish to understand how a person feels, we may adopt their posture and expression. Becoming sensitive to our inner experience, we may know exactly how that person feels.

In the same way, certain things are very difficult to explain, but must be experienced directly. Thus yogis communicate certain things by asking the student to adopt a particular posture or exercise, which itself teaches the student."

Hathapradipika

The aim of yoga is to cease the constant chitter chatter of the mind. To rid the body of toxins and accumulated bad habits so we can meditate comfortably. With practice you will learn that each posture is a meditation in itself.

Each posture should include the eight steps of Patanjali's yoga sutras, the eight fold path. Learning to incorporate these steps into just one pose, would be a lifetime's achievement. So go slowly. You do not need to learn 101 yoga postures to make progress. If you can master one pose and practice with ease, you can incorporate that knowledge and learning process into everything you do.

"Life itself is always a trial. In training you must test and polish yourself in order to face the great challenges of life. Transcend the realm of life and death, and then you will be able to make your way calmly and safely through any crisis that confronts you."

Morihei Ueshiba

Movement is guided by the breath and synchronizes with the breath. After a while we realize we are our breath. It is the breath that creates the union between the mind and the body. The movements or postures are an expression of our breath, our inner rhythm. Movement without the corresponding breathing pattern is merely exercise and is not yoga.

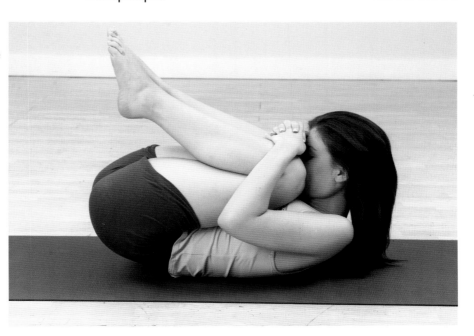

Preparation for Practice

The yoga postures can be modified and adapted to suit your needs and environment. The postures teach us to know ourselves, our limitations, our strengths, and our weaknesses. Recognizing these traits, learning to accept them, instead of fighting them, helps us to achieve perfect equilibrium and to be at peace with ourselves and our environment.

However you must find an experienced teacher who will guide you. It is important that you always inform your teacher of any injuries, illness, or disabilities. It is a good idea to commit your medical history to paper, so you can give your teacher the information needed to help you. Writing things down in a letter can avoid embarrassment in a class. Not everyone wants the whole class to know of their problems.

If you have any type of health issue, including pregnancy, you must seek your medical practitioner's consent before trying out the postures. If your doctor is unsure about yoga movements, take this book with you, emphasizing there is no strain or stress and you will be moving at your own pace. The most important things to remember are:

• Yoga should be practiced on an empty stomach, with a three-hour break from eating food. Early morning is an ideal time.

• Clothing should be loose, comfortable, and lightweight.

• You will need a yoga mat to practice on. You can use a towel or blanket, but a sticky yoga mat is best.

• Find the optimum place to practice. The room should be warm, light, and quiet.

• Make sure you will not be disturbed. Your family and friends need to get used to the idea that when you are practicing, it's time out. Our mind supplies plenty of distractions just by itself.

• Try and practice at the same time every day so you can get into a routine.

• Approach your yoga practice with grace and ease.

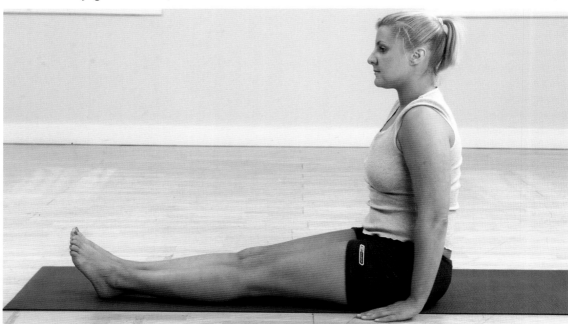

It's important to remember that yoga is for all ages and all sizes, endomorphs and ectomorphs alike.

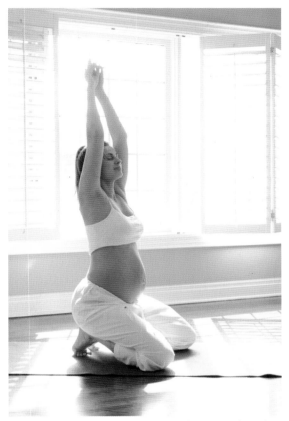

Yoga can be practiced during most weeks of pregnancy, but ask your doctor for advice.

Mothers with young children may find it difficult to practice without distractions, but you have to find the time and place to make it happen. Many people prefer to practice in the evening. In which case you must make sure your evening meal is completely digested (three hours). Include a good relaxation (at least ten minutes) at the end of the practice so you can sleep well and you are not fired up, as if you had been doing an aerobic activity.

Whatever time of day you choose to practice, it is paramount that you begin with the Complete Breath and finish with the Closing Breath. This gives us a very definite feeling of beginning and ending.

Follow instructions carefully, especially as a beginner. Know your sequence before you begin, even if it means having these written down nearby. Do not start your practice and make it up as you go along. Follow the instructions in this book and then practice and make perfect.

How to use this book

Read the instructions carefully until you are familiar with them. You may like to practice with a friend who can read the instructions out to you.

Following the breath is paramount. As you read the instructions, follow the breath and imagine yourself performing the pose. This is a great way to prepare for practice.

In time you will find you want to know more and more about yoga. On first reading this book you may find some sections too heavy or irrelevant to your needs. But with time you will be looking for more information. What may have passed you by as relatively meaningless six months ago could now be an integral part of your practice.

Practice, enjoy, and be at peace.

Before you begin

Make sure:

- The room you are practicing in is warm and light.
- You have not eaten for at least three hours.
- You have a yoga mat, or towel to practice on.
- You are wearing loose, comfortable clothing.
- You will not be disturbed.
- You have a chair or strong table near, for the modified poses.
- You are committed to a minimum of twenty minutes practice.
- You decide which sequence or postures you are going to practice, and stick with it.

The Postures
mountain pose (tadasana)

Standing still as a mountain, steady and secure. Encourages an energizing breathing pattern.

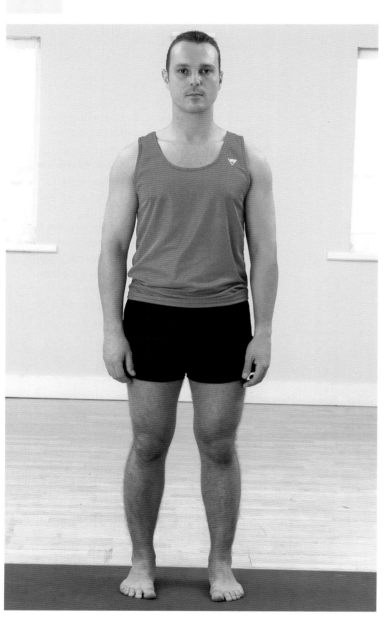

Method

1 Stand with your feet hip width apart.

2 Keep your eyes forward, spine erect, and arms by your sides.

3 Distribute your weight evenly along the length of your feet.

4 Listen to your breathing.

5 Breathe in, fill, and expand your lungs.

6 Breathe out, contract, and empty your lungs.

7 Make at least four complete breaths, until your breathing becomes smooth and rhythmic.

8 Tune into the rhythm of your breath. Focus your attention on your breath.

9 Become aware of the rise of your chest as you breathe in, the fall of your chest as you breathe out.

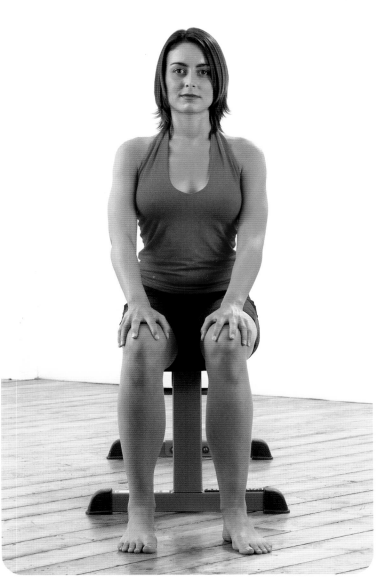

Benefits

- Masters the art of standing correctly, in correct alignment.
- Develops stability and an awareness of your posture.
- Provides a foundation from which other postures are developed.
- Corrects imbalances in the posture, breath, and flow of energy.
- Calms the breath.

Precautions

- Don't tense your spine. The knees should be soft, not locked.

Modification
1 Sit on a straight-backed, armless chair, with your feet flat on the floor and palms resting on your thighs.
2 Keep your spine erect and your eyes forward.
3 Breathe normally.

complete breath

Helps to harmonize the breath and movement. Energizes the body and mind.

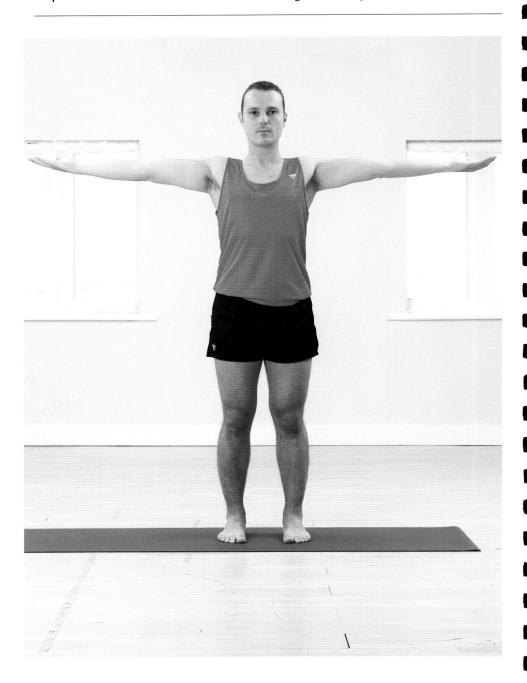

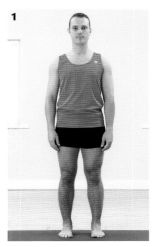

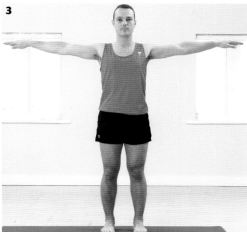

Benefits

- Energizes the entire system, overcoming fatigue.
- Increases the intake of oxygen, resulting in clarity of mind and a healthy, glowing complexion.

Precautions

- Don't force your breath.
- Remember, the movement follows your breath.

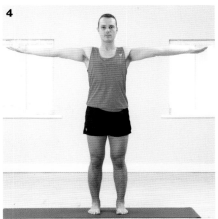

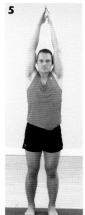

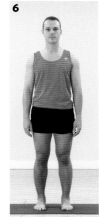

Method

1 Stand in Mountain Pose.

2 Breathe in and out.

3 Breathe in, raise your arms to shoulder level.

4 Breathe out, turn your palms to the sky.

5 Breathe in, raise your arms above your head, palms facing each other.

6 Breathe out, lower you arms to your sides.

7 Allow your breath to guide your movements.

8 Repeat four times.

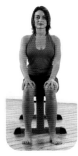

Modification
- This posture can be practiced either sitting on a chair or lying supine on the floor.

refresher breath/moon pose

Encourages the mind and body to relax.

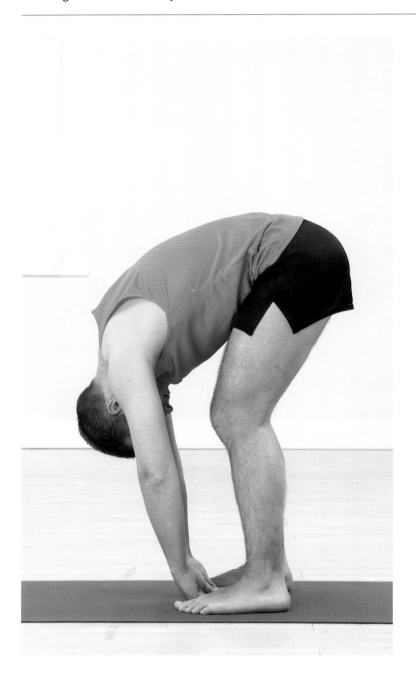

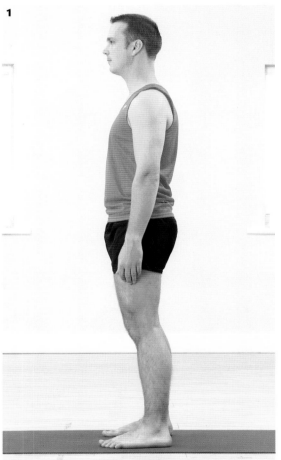

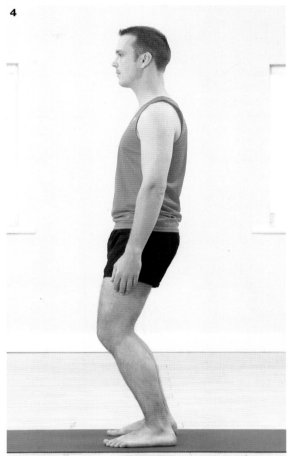

Method

1 Stand in Mountain Pose.
2 Breathe in and out.
3 Breathe in.
4 Breathe out, bend your knees.
5 Breathe in.

refresher breath/moon pose (continued)

6 Breathe out. Let your chin fall toward your chest.

7 Breathe in.

8 Breathe out and let your body fold forward, bending at the hips, and relaxing toward the floor.

9 Breathe in. Look between your thighs.

10 Breathe out.

11 Breathe in and out.

12 Breathe in. Slowly uncurl, vertebra by vertebra. Come up to standing. Your head comes up last.

13 Breathe out. Keep your eyes forward.

14 Repeat four times.

15 The movement follows your breath.

6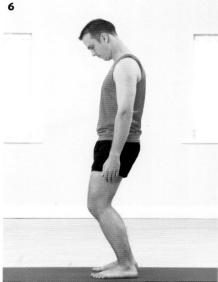

8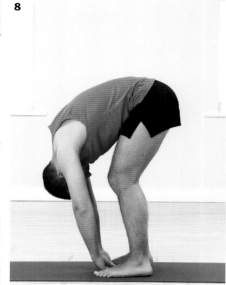

12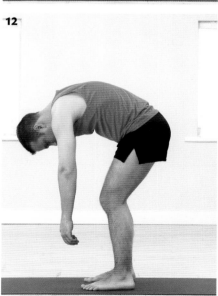

13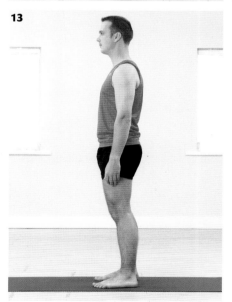

Benefits

- Gently stretches the lower back and the back of the legs.
- Relaxes the neck, shoulders, arms, and hands.
- Blood flows into the head to refresh and revitalize.

Precautions

- Only relax forward as far as you comfortably can. There should be no pain.
- If you suffer from high blood pressure, heart disease, glaucoma, detached retina, or back pain practice the modified pose.

Modifications

1 Place a strong chair or table an arm's length away from you to the front.
2 Breath in.
3 Breathe out. Relax forward, place your hands on the back of the chair.
4 Lengthen your spine. Look to the floor, with your knees bent.
5 Breathe in and out three times.
6 Breathe in as you come up to standing.
7 Breathe out. Relax.
8 Repeat four times, then breathe normally.

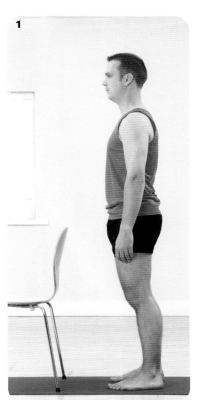

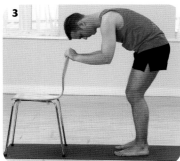

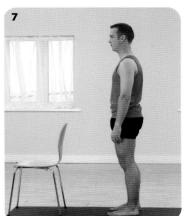

27

abdominal lift

Drawing the belly towards your spine. Slims and tones the whole of the abdominal area.
Stimulates the fire energy.

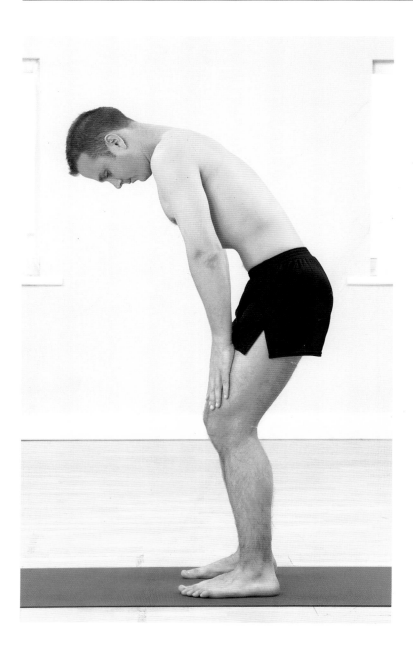

1

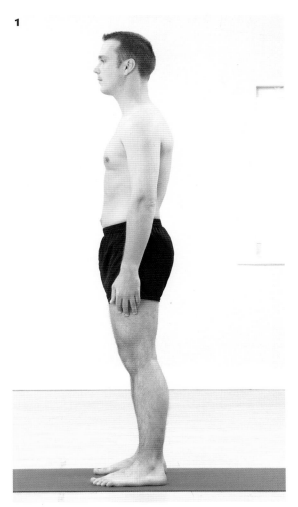

8

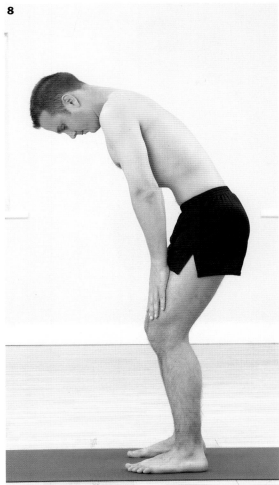

Method

1 Stand in Mountain Pose

2 Breathe in and out.

3 Breathe in.

4 Breathe out. Bend your knees.

5 Breathe in.

6 Breathe out. Lean forwards, place your palms onto your thighs.

7 Gently rounding your back, keep your elbows away from your sides.

8 Breathe in and fill your lungs.

abdominal lift (continued)

14

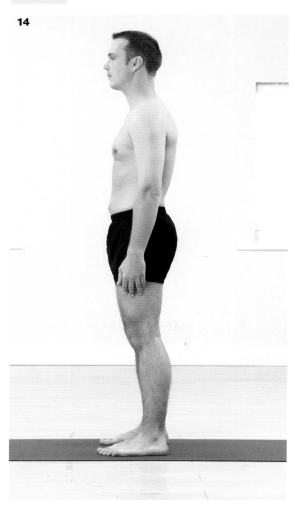

9 Breathe out. Draw your belly towards your spine.

10 Squeeze your ribs together.

11 Draw your belly inward and upward.

12 Look between your thighs.

13 Hold the pose, then relax your belly.

14 Come up to standing with your spine erect and eyes forward. Breathe in.

15 Breathe out and bring your arms to your sides.

16 Repeat four times, then breathe easy.

Benefits

- Tones and slims the abdominal area. The waist becomes slimmer.
- Helps to tighten up the pelvic floor.
- Increases strength and flexibility in the abdomen.
- Helps eliminate toxins in the digestive tract.
- Increases awareness of the movement of the diaphragm as we breathe in and out.
- Increases the quality of the breath.

Precautions

- Don't force your breath.
- Avoid this posture if you are menstruating, have inflammation in the abdominal areas or suffer from high blood pressure.

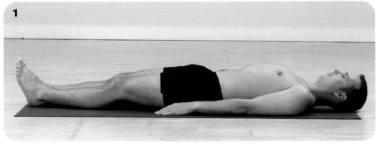

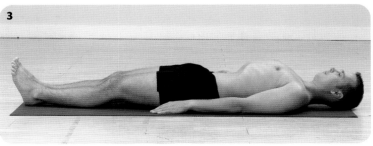

Modification

1 Lie supine on the floor.

2 Breathe in. Expand and fill your lungs.

3 Breathe out. Draw your stomach towards your spine. Squeeze your ribs together. Draw your stomach inward and upward. Keep your eyes looking at the ceiling. Hold the pose.

4 Then relax your belly. Breathe in and out.

5 Repeat four times.

6 Breathe in. Roll yourself over and up to a seated pose

7 Breathe out. Breathe normally.

sun salutation standing

Opens energy centers and improves the posture. A harmony in breath and movement.

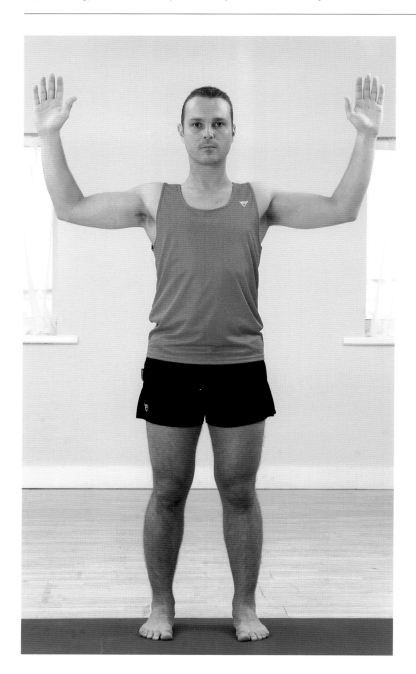

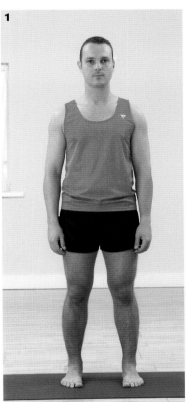

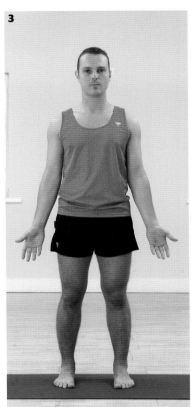

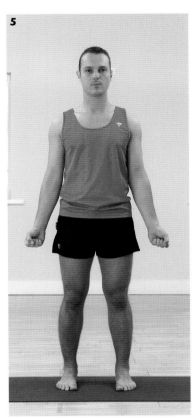

Method

1 Stand in Mountain Pose.

2 Breathe in and out.

3 Breathe in. Turn your palms to face the front.

4 Breathe out.

5 Breathe in. Lightly clench your hands into fists.

sun salutation standing (continued)

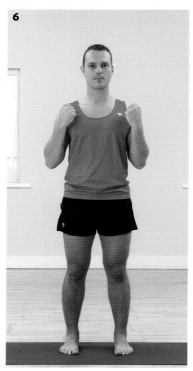

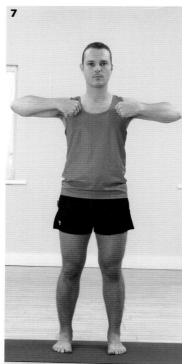

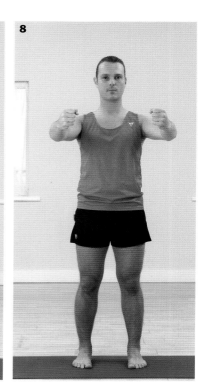

6 Breathe out. Raise your fists to your shoulders.

7 Breathe in. Raise your elbows.

8 Breathe out and stretch out your arms in front of you, keeping them at shoulder level.

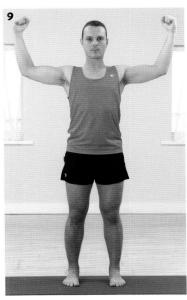

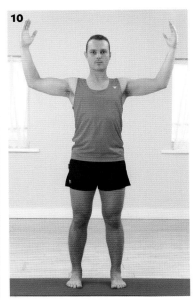

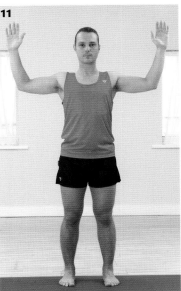

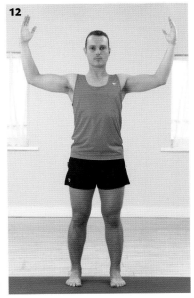

9 Breathe in. Raise your hands, keeping your elbows at shoulder level.

10 Breathe out. Turn your palms to face each other.

11 Breathe in and turn your palms to face forward.

12 Breathe out. Turn your palms to face each other.

sun salutation standing (continued)

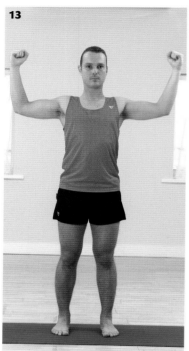

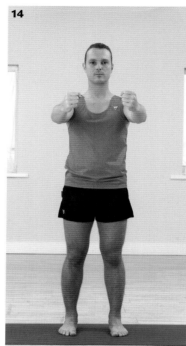

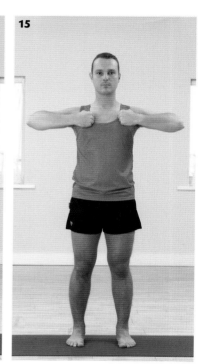

13 Breathe in and lightly clench
   your hands.

14 Breathe out and stretch out your
   arms in front of you, keeping
   them at shoulder level.

15 Breathe in. Bring your fists in to
   your shoulders.

16 Breathe out. Lower your elbows.

17 Breathe in. Lower your arms.

18 Breathe out. Open your palms.

19 Breathe normally in
   Mountain Pose.

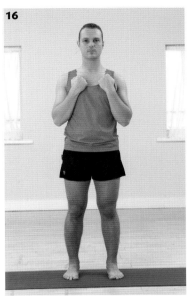

16

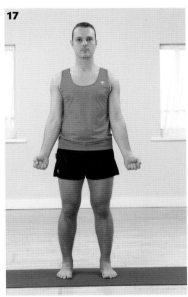

17

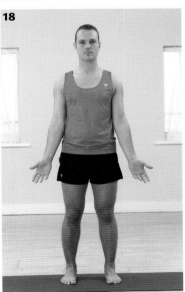

18

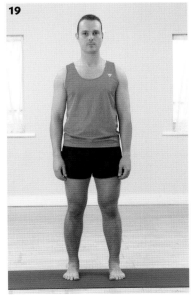

19

Benefits

- Encourages a deep, rhythmic breathing pattern.
- Opens and stimulates energy centers that are connected to the healthy functioning of the internal organs.
- Increases vitality and aids concentration.
- Helps calm the emotions.

Precautions

- Take your time and do not rush this posture. Keep your shoulders away from your ears (i.e. not hunched up).
- Follow the natural rhythm of your breath.

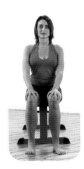

Modification
- Sit on a straight-backed chair and follow the instructions as above.

37

standing forward bend 1

A pose where you bring your hands to your feet or ankles. It helps clear and calm the mind.

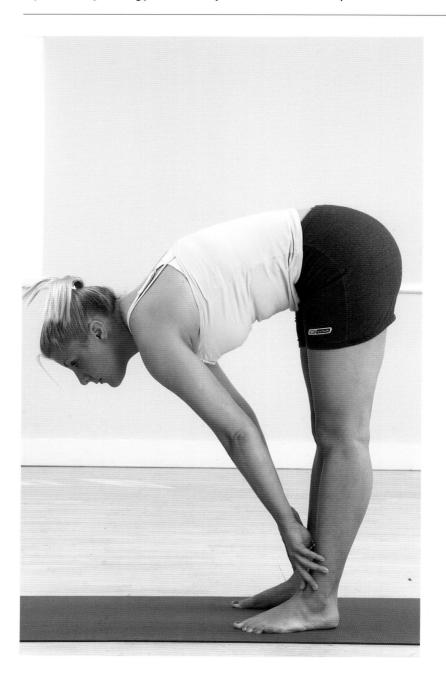

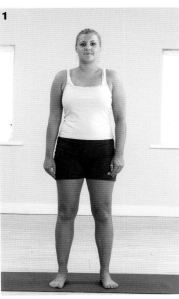

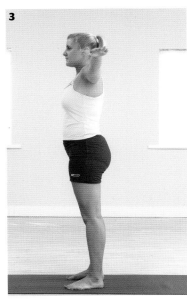

Method:

1 Stand in Mountain Pose.

2 Breathe in and out.

3 Breathe in. Raise your arms to shoulder level.

4 Breathe out. Place your hands on your hips.

5 Breathe in. Lift up through your waist.

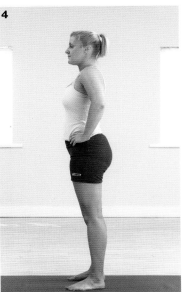

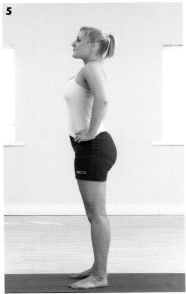

standing forward bend 1 (continued)

6　Breathe out. Relax forwards, bending and rolling over the hips. Leading out with the chest, then chin, nose, eyes, forehead, and the top of your head toward the floor. Look between your thighs.

7　Breathe in.

8　Breathe out. Slide your hands down your legs, elbows bent, resting your hands on your legs, where you can hold the pose comfortably. Hold the pose.

9　Breathe in and out three times.

10　Breathe in. Look forward.

11　Breathe out. Place your hands onto your hips.

12　Breathe in. Lift up through your waist.

13　Come up to standing with your eyes forward and spine erect.

14　Breathe out and bring your arms to your sides.

15　Repeat four times.

16　Breathe normally.

Enjoy the release of tension in the spine and mind. Once you have gained sufficient flexibility, progress to Forward Bends 2 and 3.

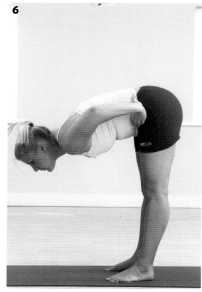

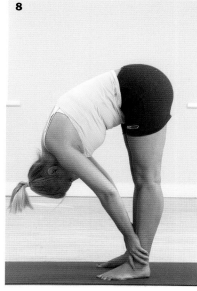

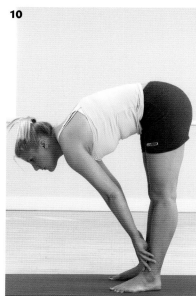

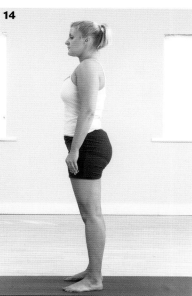

Benefits

- Slims and firms the arms, waist, abdomen, buttocks, and legs.
- Promotes a youthful vigor.
- Lengthens the spine, increasing its flexibility.
- Stretches all the muscles of the back of the body.
- Creates a foundation from which other forward bends are developed.
- Can correct a small imbalance in the length of the legs.
- Aids concentration.
- Invigorates the entire nervous system.
- Increases the circulation to the legs, torso, and brain.
- Massages the internal organs.

Precautions

- If you suffer from high blood pressure, do not lower your head below your heart. Practice the modified pose.
- If your hamstrings are tight, do not cause yourself discomfort or pain.
- If you have a slipped disk, do not do it. Accept your body's limitations.
- Keep your weight in the front of your feet, do not push into your heels.

Modification

1 Keep your knees soft, not locked.
2 Breathe in. Lift up through your waist.
3 Breathe out. Fold forward, place your palms onto your thighs, with your eyes to the floor. Focus on lengthening your spine. Hold the pose.
4 Breathe in and out three times
5 Breathe in. Look forward and come up to a standing position.
6 Breathe out. Place your arms at your sides.
7 Repeat four times.
8 Breathe normally.
9 Stand in Mountain Pose.

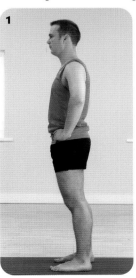
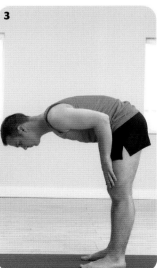
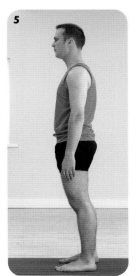
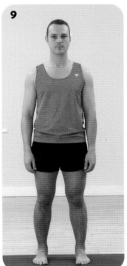

standing forward bend 2

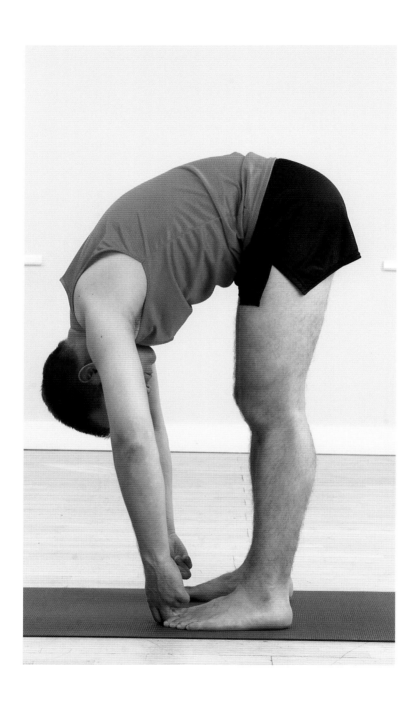

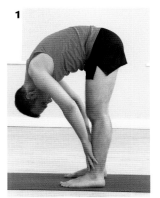
1

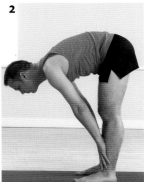
2

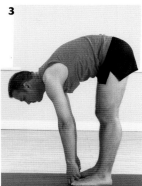
3

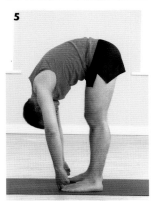
5

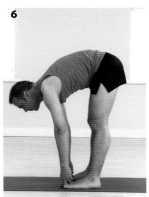
6

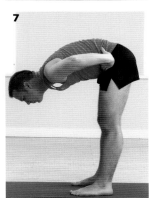
7

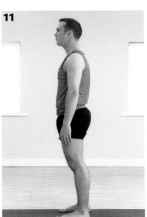
11

Method

1 Continue from Standing Forward Bend 1(Pic 8), with your hands resting on your legs.

2 Breathe in. Look forward.

3 Breathe out. Hook your first two fingers under each big toe.

4 Breathe in. Draw up on the back of your legs.

5 Breathe out. Bend your elbows. Try to get your chest to your thighs. Look between your thighs. Hold the pose and breathe in and out three times.

6 Breathe in. Look forwards.

7 Breathe out. Hands onto your hips.

8 Breathe in. Come up to standing with your eyes forward and spine erect.

9 Breathe out. Bring your arms to your sides.

10 Breathe easy.

11 Stand in Mountain Pose.

standing forward bend 3

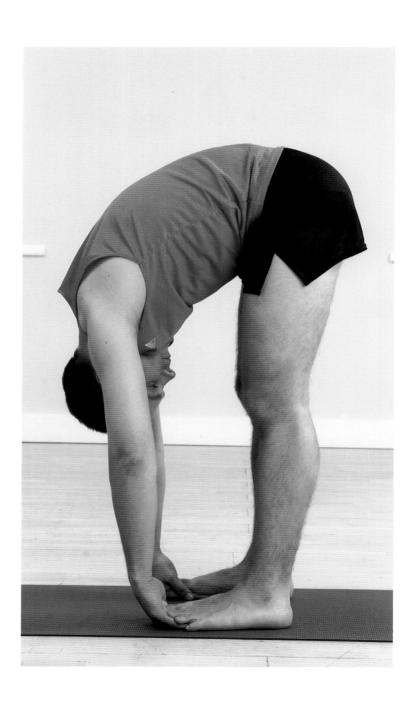

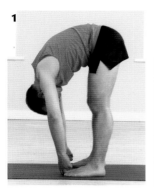

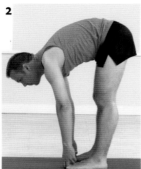

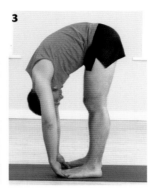

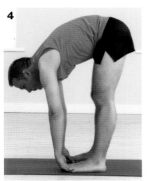

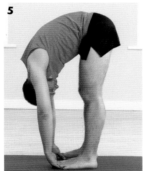

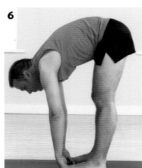

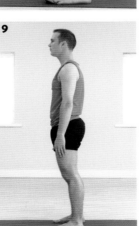

Method

1 Continue from Standing Forward Bend 2 (Pic 5).

2 Breathe in. Look forwards.

3 Breathe out. Place your palms under the soles of your feet.

4 Breathe in. Look forward.

5 Breathe out. Bend your elbows. Try to bring your chest to your thighs and look between them. Hold the pose. Breathe in and out three times.

6 Breathe in. Look forwards.

7 Breathe out. Bring your hands to your hips.

8 Breathe in. Come up to standing.

9 Breathe out. Bring your arms to your sides. Keep your spine erect and your eyes forward. Breathe normally.

standing back bend

By arching your spine in the opposite direction this posture acts as a contrapose to the forward bends described earlier.

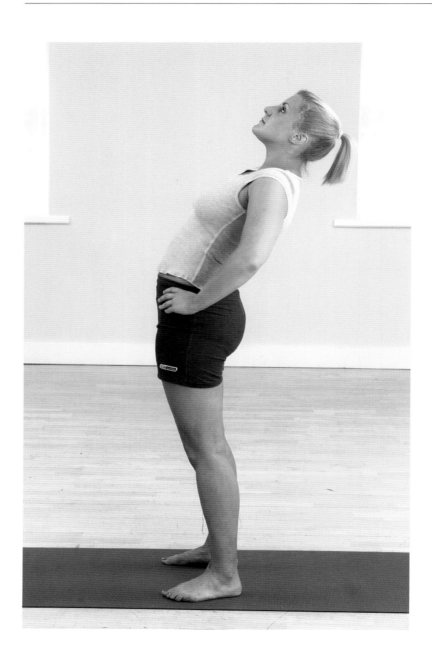

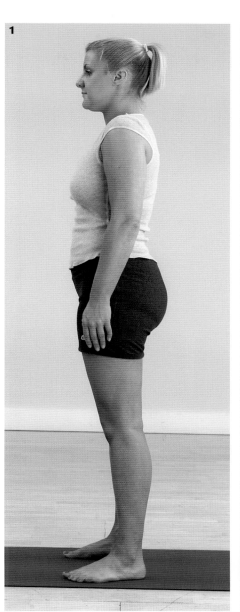

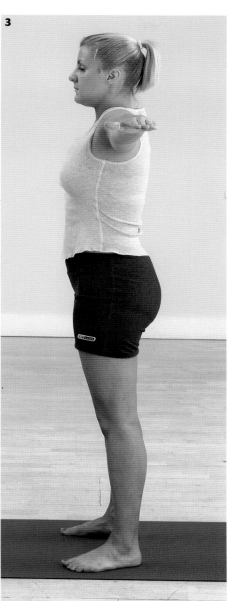

Method

1 Stand in
   Mountain Pose.

2 Breathe in
   and out.

3 Breathe in.
   Raise your arms
   at your sides to
   shoulder level.

standing back bend (continued)

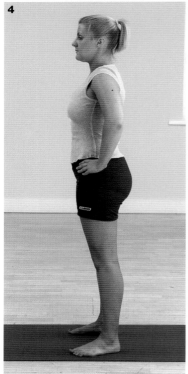 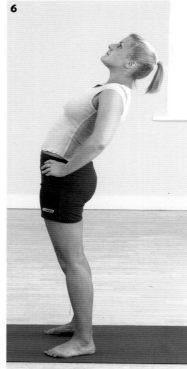 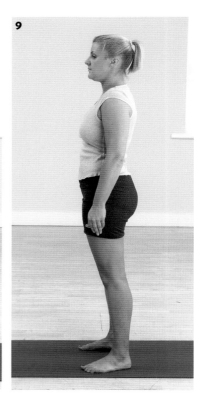

4   Breathe out. Place your hands on your hips.

5   Breathe in. Lift up through your waist.

6   Breathe out. Gently arch your spine. Raising your chest to the ceiling, eyes to the ceiling also.

7   Breathe in and out three times.

8   Breathe in.

9   Breathe out. Lower your chest, face, and eyes.

10 Breathe in. Keep your eyes forward and your spine erect.

11 Breathe out. Lower your arms to your sides.

12 Breathe normally. Be aware of tension, release it and let it go.

Benefits

- Releases tension in the lower back.
- Helps to slim the waist.
- Tones and stretches the neck and refreshes the face.
- Strengthens the spine and increases the flexibility of the spine.

Precautions

- Only go as far as is comfortable. If in doubt, leave it out.

Modification

1 Place both hands on your lower back, fingers pointing toward your buttocks.
2 Massage this area with your hands.
3 Make nine circles in each direction.
4 Relax.

■ *Helps to relieve tension and any discomfort.*

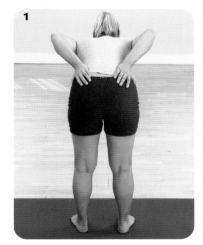

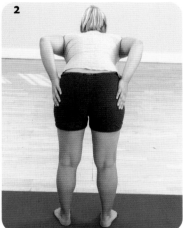

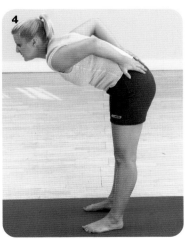

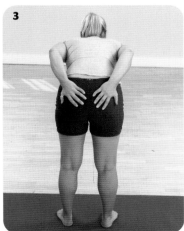

triangle pose (trikonasana)

Extend to the right and left in this pose. Triangle Pose helps to tone, slim, and shape the waist and legs. It builds strength and flexibility in the legs.

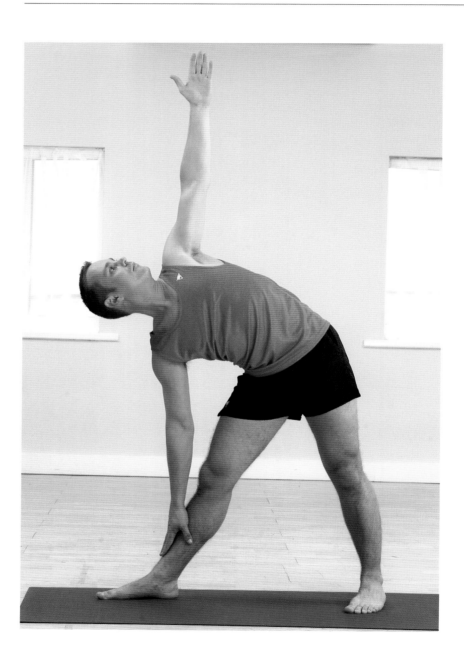

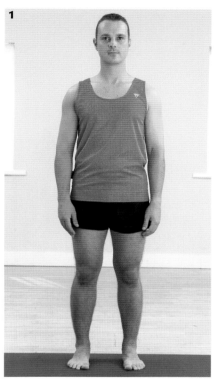

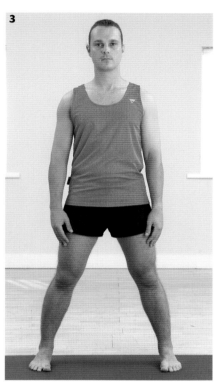

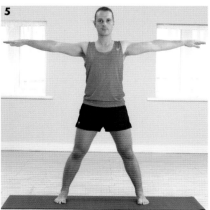

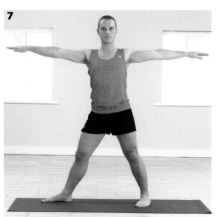

Method

1 Stand in Mountain Pose.

2 Breathe normally.

3 Walk your feet, double hip width apart. Keep your feet parallel and your eyes forward.

4 Breathe in and out.

5 Breathe in. Raise your arms to shoulder level.

6 Breathe out. Turn your left foot inward 45 degrees. Your left big toe points toward your right big toe.

7 Breathe in. Turn your right foot 90 degrees to the right.

triangle pose (trikonasana) (continued)

8 Breathe out. Relax. Check your pose for comfort and ease.

9 Breathe in. Lift up through the waist. Reach out to the right.

10 Breathe out. Bend to the right, placing your hand on the outside of your lower leg.

11 Breathe in. Look up toward your raised hand.

12 Breathe out. Extend your raised arm to the sky. Hold the pose.

13 Breathe in and out three times.

14 Breathe in. Lift up through your waist, come up to standing, keeping your arms parallel to the floor and your spine erect.

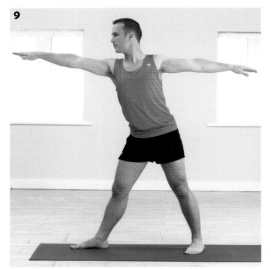

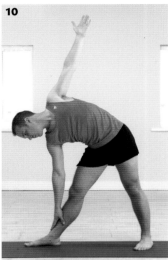

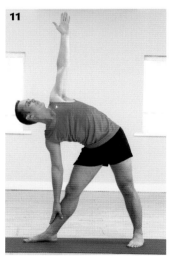

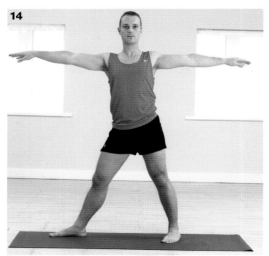

16

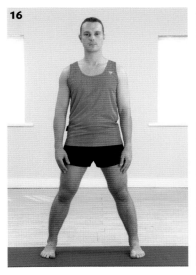

20

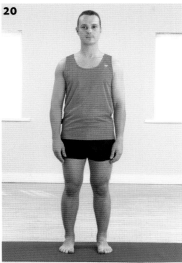

15 Breathe out and move your arms to your sides. Breathe in. Turn your feet back to face the front.

16 Breathe out. Keep your eyes forward.

17 Breathe in and out

18 Repeat to the opposite side.

19 Walk your feet back to hip width apart.

20 Stand in Mountain Pose.

21 Breathe normally.

Benefits

- Stretches, slims, and tones the waist, hips, and thighs.
- An invigorating stretch which makes the whole body feel lighter.
- Stimulates the circulation.
- Opens and develops the chest, building strength and stamina.
- Increases flexibility.
- Aids digestion and helps regulate the appetite.

Precautions

- Only go as far as you comfortably can. If you have back problems, place your hand on your thigh and not on your lower leg.
- If you have neck problems, do not turn your head to look at your raised hand and keep your eyes looking forward.
- Do not overstretch, it will work against you.
- Do not bend your raised arm.
- Distribute your weight evenly, between each leg and foot.
- Do not sink into your hips.

Modification
- If you have neck problems, do not turn your head to look at your raised hand and keep your eyes looking forward.
- Bend your knee when coming up to a standing position.

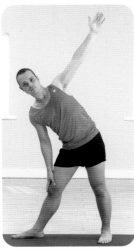

53

legs wide forward bend 1 (prasarita padottanasana)

This pose will significantly stretch the legs and is expanding, extending, and rejuvenating.

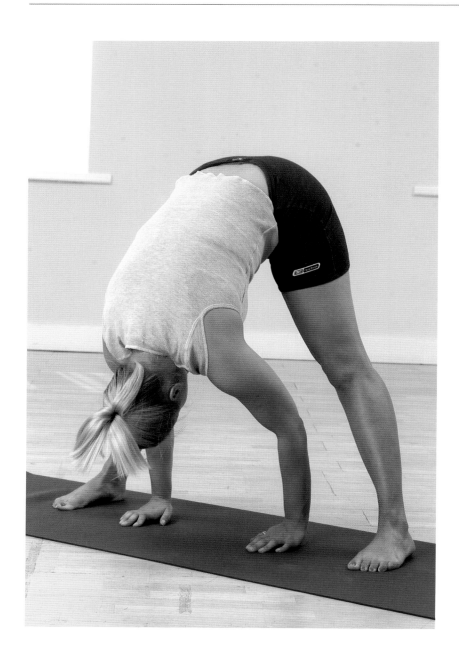

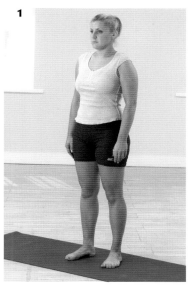

1

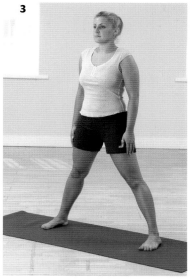

3

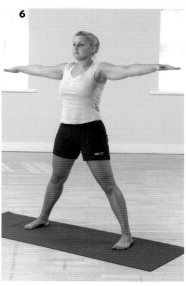

6

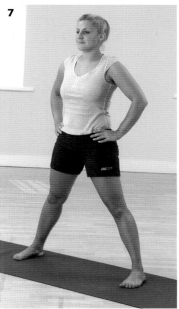

7

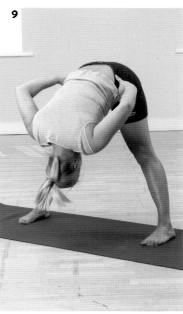

9

Method

1 Stand in Mountain Pose.

2 Breathe easy.

3 Walk your feet to double hip width apart.

4 Keep your feet parallel and your eyes forward.

5 Breathe in and out.

6 Breathe in. Raise your arms to shoulder level.

7 Breathe out. Place your hands on your hips.

8 Breathe in. Lift up through your waist.

9 Breathe out. Bend at your hips. Reach forward and relax downward with the top of your head toward the floor. Look between your thighs.

legs wide forward bend 1 (continued)

10 Breathe in. Place your palms flat on the floor with your fingers parallel to your toes.

11 Breathe out. Let the top of your head relax toward the floor. Breathe in and out three times.

12 Breathe in. Look forward.

13 Breathe out. Move your hands onto your hips.

14 Breathe in. Lift up through your waist, come up to standing with your eyes forward and spine erect.

15 Breathe out and bring your arms to your sides.

16 Breathe normally.

17 Feel the stretch on the back of your legs.

18 Walk your feet back to hip width apart.

19 Stand in Mountain Pose.

10
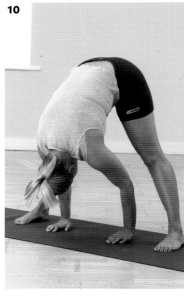

12
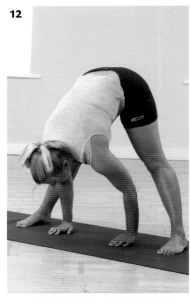

13
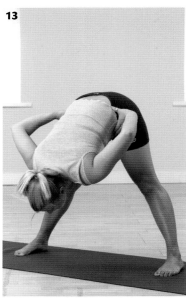

15
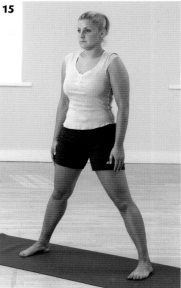

Benefits

- Tones and firms the back of the legs and especially the thighs.
- Increases the flow of blood to the brain.
- Relieves headaches, anxiety, irritability, and insomnia.
- Aids the digestive process.

Precautions

- For those with back problems, keep your knees bent.
- If you have a heart condition, high blood pressure, detached retina, or glaucoma, practice the modified pose.
- Keep your legs firm and draw up on the back of your knees. Make sure the backs of your knees are soft, not locked.

Modification

1 Follow the instructions for Legs Wide Forward Bend 1 until you place your hands on your hips.
2 Breathe in. Lift up through your waist.
3 Breathe out. Bend forward at the hips, keeping your spine long, eyes to the floor, and chest parallel to the floor. Hold the pose.
4 Breathe in and out three times.
5 Breathe in. Lift up through your waist. Come up to a standing position.
6 Breathe out. Bring your arms to your sides and your eyes forward.

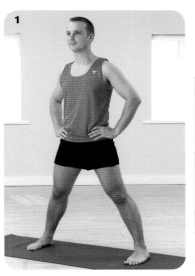
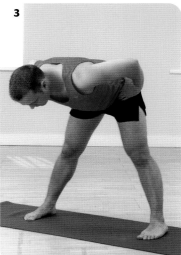
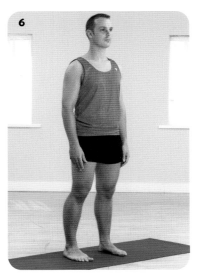

legs wide forward bend 2

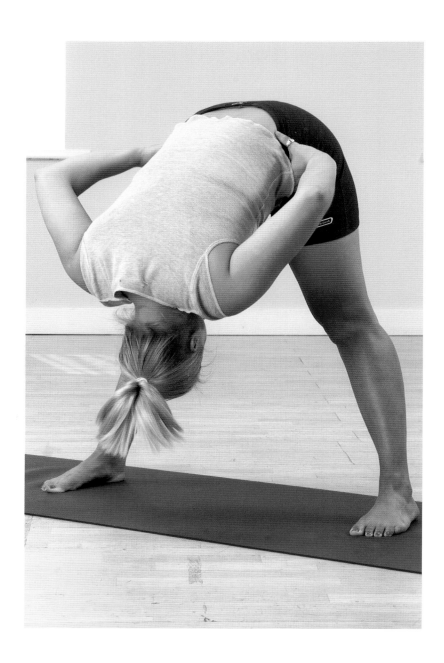

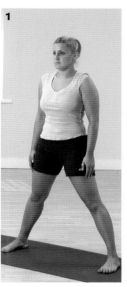

1

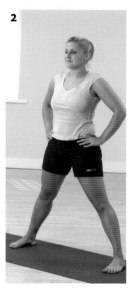

2

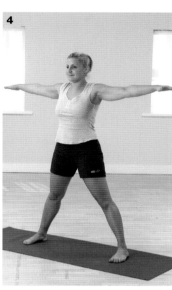

4

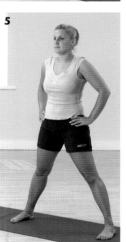

5

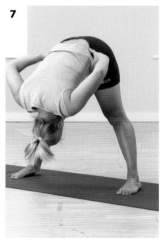

7

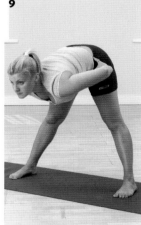

9

Method

1 Start with your legs double hip width apart.

2 Place your hands on your hips.

3 Breathe in and out.

4 Breathe in. Raise your arms to shoulder level.

5 Breathe out. Move your hands to your hips again.

6 Breathe in. Lift up through your waist.

7 Breathe out. Bend at the hips, reach forward, relax downward, with the top of your head toward the floor. Look between your thighs.

8 Breathe in and out three times.

9 Breathe in. Look forward.

10 Breathe out.

11 Breathe in. Lift up through your waist. Come up to standing with your eyes forward and your spine erect.

12 Breathe out with your arms to your sides.

13 Breathe normally.

legs wide forward bend 3

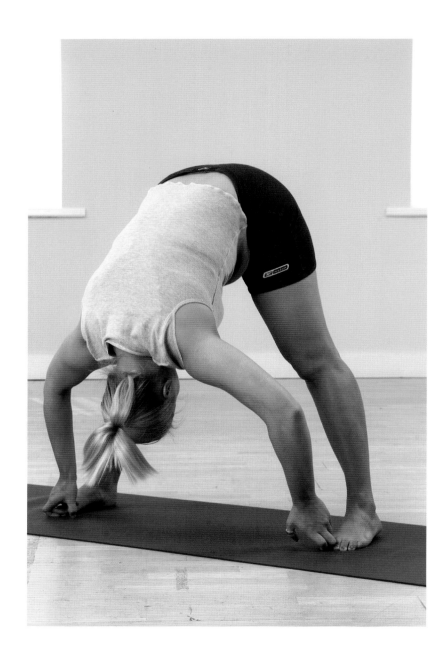

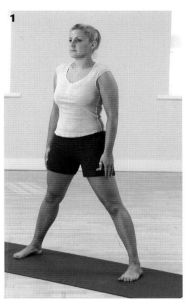

1

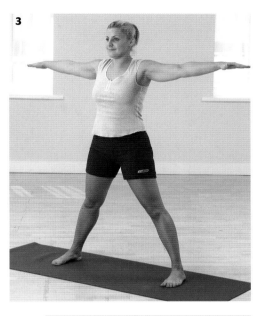

3

Method

1 Place your feet double hip width apart.

2 Breathe in and out.

3 Breathe in. Raise your arms to shoulder level.

4 Breathe out. Place your hands on your hips.

5 Breathe in. Lift up through your waist.

6 Breathe out. Bend at the hips and reach forward, relaxing downward with the top of your head toward the floor. Look between your thighs.

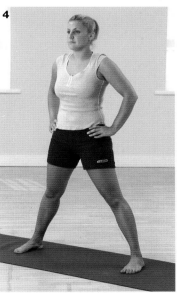

4

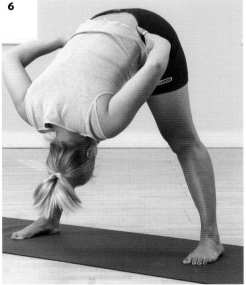

6

legs wide forward bend 3 (continued)

7 Breathe in.
  Look forward.

8 Hook your first
  two fingers under
  each big toe.

9 Breathe out. Bend
  your elbows and
  chest toward your
  thighs. Draw the
  top of your head
  down toward the
  floor. Look between
  your thighs.
  Hold the pose.

10 Breathe in and
   out three times.

11 Breathe in.
   Look forward.

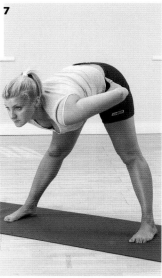

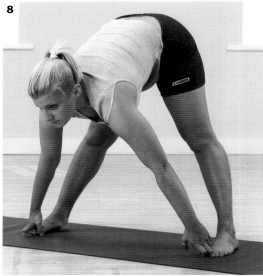

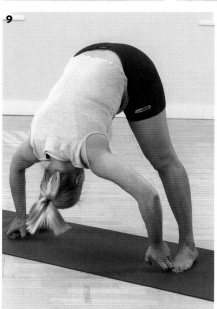

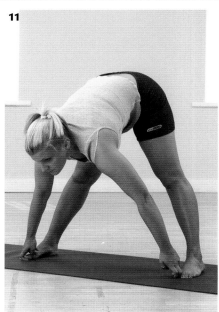

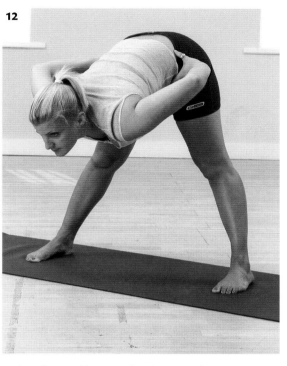

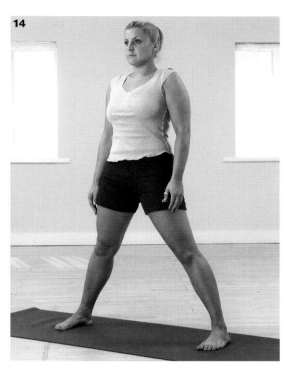

12 Breathe out. Place your hands on your hips.

13 Breathe in. Lift up through your waist, come up to standing position with your eyes forward and spine erect.

14 Breathe out with arms to your sides.

15 Breathe normally.

16 Walk your feet back to hip width apart and stand in Mountain Pose.

warrior, pose 1 (virabhadrasana)

This is a very dynamic posture that tones, slims, and strengthens nearly all parts of the body. It cultivates a strong body and healthy mind.

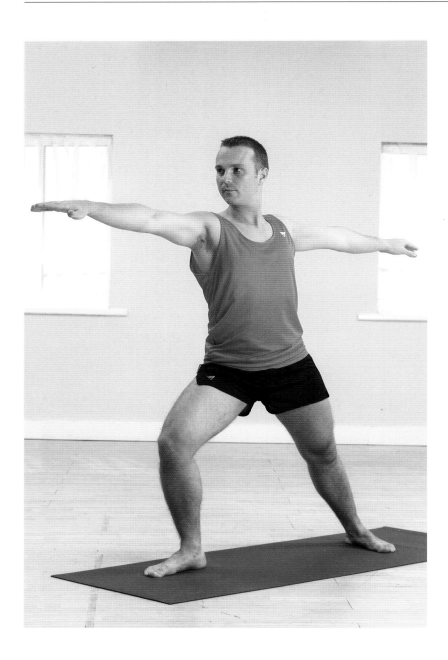

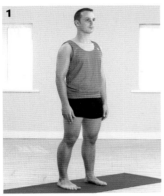
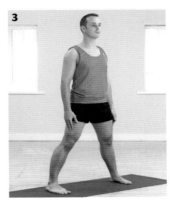
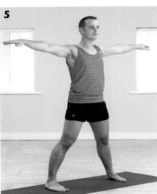
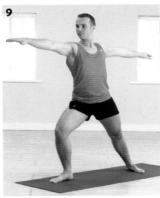
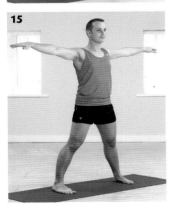
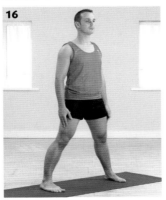

Method

1 Stand in Mountain Pose.

2 Breathe normally.

3 Walk your feet double hip width apart, with your feet parallel and your eyes forward.

4 Breathe in and out.

5 Breathe in. Raise your arms to shoulder level.

6 Breathe out. Imagine your arms resting on clouds.

7 Breathe in. Turn your right foot 90 degrees away from you.

8 Breathe out. Bend your right knee, so that the knee is directly above your toes.

9 Breathe in. Look along the fingertips of your right hand.

10 Open your chest.

11 Extend out through your fingertips.

12 Breathe out. Press the outside edge of your back foot flat to the floor.

13 Breathe in and out three times.

14 Breathe in. Straighten your right leg.

15 Breathe out. Turn your right foot back to face the front.

16 Move your arms to your sides.

17 Breathe normally.

18 Repeat to your left side.

19 Feel your inner strength and balance.

20 Walk your feet back to hip width apart. Stand in Mountain Pose.

warrior, pose 2

This pose specifically reduces fat around the hips.

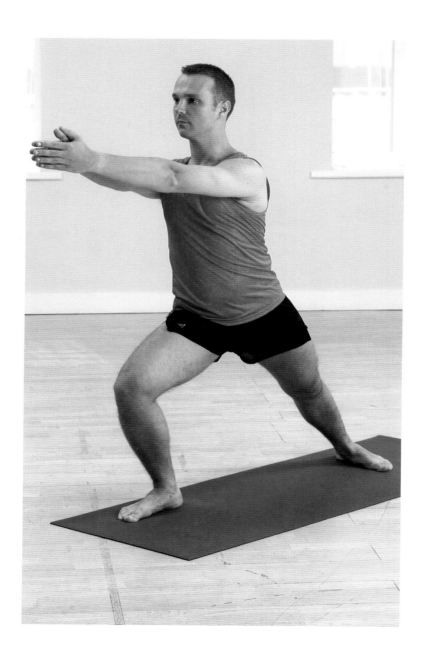

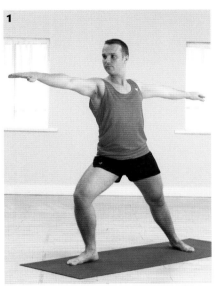

1

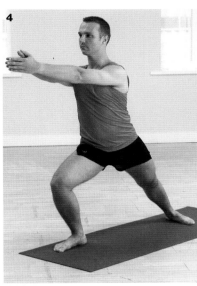

4

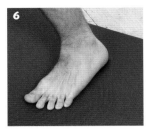

6

Method

1 Start at Warrior Pose 1.

2 Breathe in and out.

3 Breathe in. Bring your left arm forward, parallel to your right arm.

4 Breathe out. Place your palms together.

5 Breathe in. Extend through your fingertips.

6 Breathe out. Press the outside of your back foot flat to the floor.

7 Breathe in and out three times.

8 Breathe in. Return to Warrior Pose 1 with your arms parallel to the floor.

9 Breathe out. Breathe in. Turn your right foot 90 degrees back to face the front. Look forward.

10 Breathe out. Place your arms by your sides. Breathe normally.

11 Repeat to your left side.

12 Walk your feet back to hip width apart.

13 Stand in Mountain Pose.

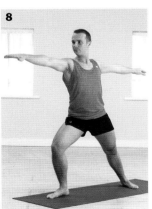

8

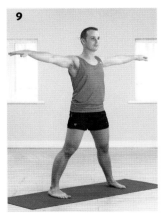

9

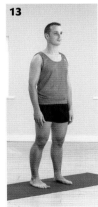

13

warrior, pose 3

This pose reduces fat around the waist, hips, back, and upper arms.

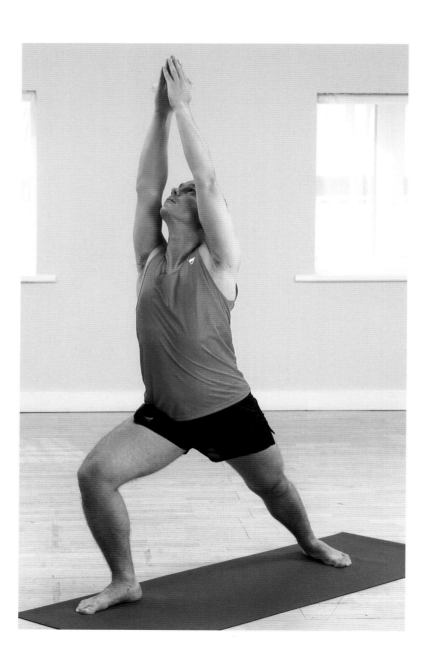

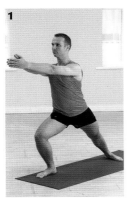

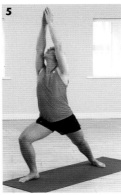

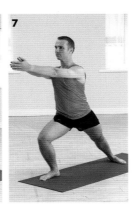

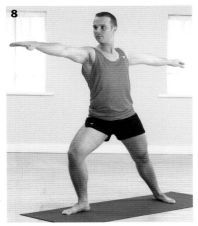

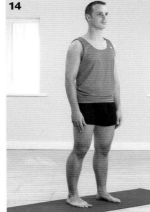

12 Breathe easy.

13 Repeat to your left side.

14 Walk your feet back to hip width apart.

15 Stand in Mountain Pose.

Benefits

- Reduces fat around the waist and hips, back and upper arms.
- Strengthens and slims the back of the legs and ankles.
- Develops deep breathing.
- Relieves stiffness in the back, neck, and shoulders.
- Tones and strengthens the abdominal organs.
- Enhances balance, poise, and inner strength.

■ *With practice and perseverance one arrives at a feeling of harmony and peace.*

Precautions

- If you have back problems, move slowly with mindful awareness.
- If you have high blood pressure or a heart condition, hold the pose only for as long as it remains comfortable to do so.

Modification

- If this pose proves too strenuous or seems too difficult, stand in Mountain Pose and cultivate the mind of a warrior. Find strength, valor, and vigor within yourself. Imagine yourself as a fearless warrior. And then, try the pose again.

Method

1 Start from Warrior Pose 2.

2 Breathe in and out.

3 Breathe in. Raise your arms above your head.

4 Breathe out. Sink your hips.

5 Breathe in. Look at your fingertips. Lift your chest up. Settle into the posture and hold.

6 Breathe in and out three times.

7 Breathe in. Return to the Warrior Pose 2 position.

8 Bring your left arm to your left side.

9 Breathe out. Turn your right foot back to face the front.

10 Breathe in. Look forward.

11 Breathe out. Lower your arms to your sides.

downward dog (adho mukha svanasana)

An exhilarating posture that strengthens and shapes the legs and arms.

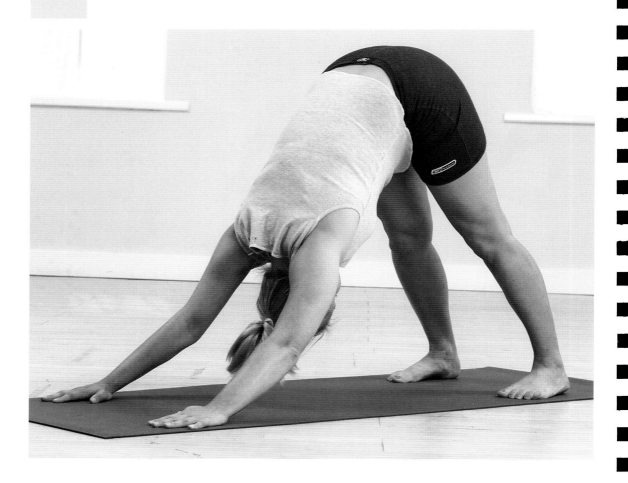

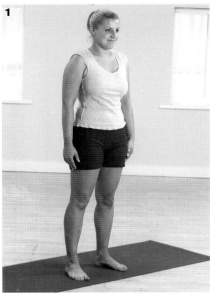

1

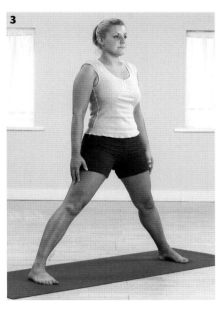

3

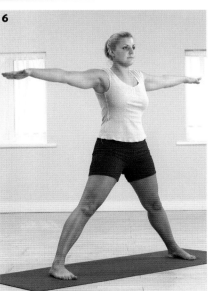

6

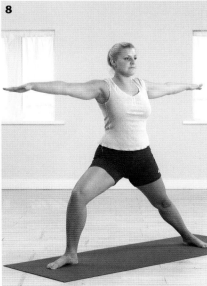

8

Method

1 Stand in Mountain Pose.

2 Breathe normally.

3 Walk your feet to double hip width apart.

4 Keep your eyes forward and your spine erect.

5 Breathe in and out.

6 Breathe in. Raise your arms to shoulder level.

7 Breathe out. Imagine your arms resting on clouds.

8 Breathe in. Turn your right foot 90 degrees away from you.

downward dog (continued)

9   Breathe out. Bend your right knee.

10 Breathe in. Bring your left arm forward, parallel to the right arm. Palms face downward.

11 Breathe out. Place your palms flat to the floor, either side of your right foot.

12 Look between your thighs.

13 Breathe in. Pivot on the ball of your left foot, turning the heel away from you, so your toes point toward your fingers.

14 Breathe out. Step back with your right foot. Keep your feet flat on the floor and hip width apart. Your heels should lengthen toward the floor.

15 Breathe in. Draw up on the back of your legs. Point the bottom of your spine, your tail bone, to the ceiling with your hips lifted.

16 Breathe out. Look toward your navel. Keep your shoulders away from your ears.

17 Breathe in and out three times.

18 Draw your shoulder blades together. Feel them lengthening down your back. Hold the pose.

19 Breathe normally.

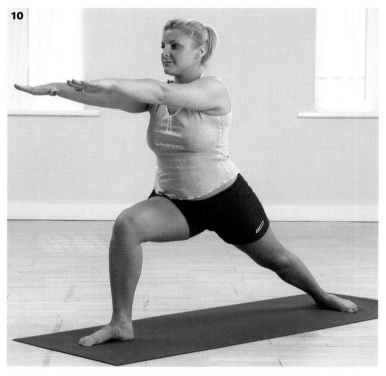

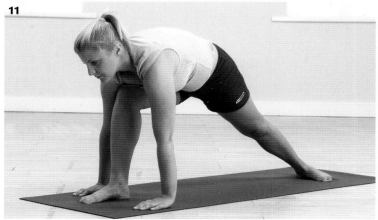

13

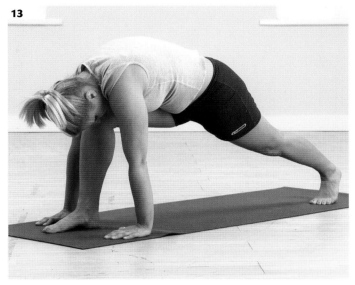

Benefits

- Firms, tones, and strengthens the arms, shoulders, spine, and abdominal areas.
- Helps combat fatigue.
- Stimulates the flow of vital energy.
- Relieves stiffness in the ankles and heels, the back of the legs, and the shoulders.
- Makes the legs shapely and slows the heartbeat.

Precautions

- If you have a back problem, keep your knees bent throughout this posture.
- Don't hunch your shoulders up around your ears.
- To help you in this pose, imagine a line of energy running from the very base of your spine, along your spine, down your arms, and out through your fingertips.

15

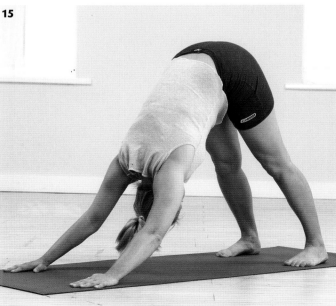

Modification
- If this posture is difficult to achieve, walk your feet closer toward your hands until you can get your heels onto or close to the floor.
- Bend your knees.
- With practice this becomes a real pose to relax and rejuvenate in.

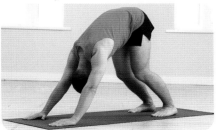

73

swan pose

A relaxing pose that stretches the arms and shoulders, and tones the upper arms.

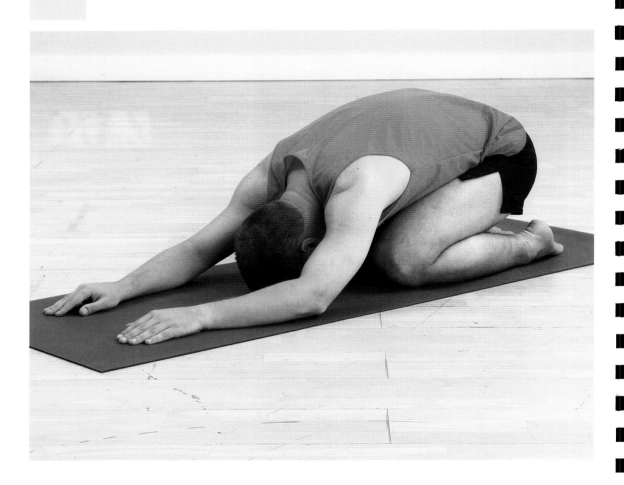

1

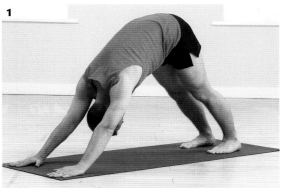

3

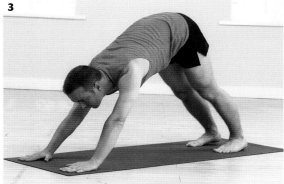

Method

1   Start in Downward Dog.

2   Breathe in and out.

3   Breathe in. Look forward.

4   Breathe out. Bend your knees and then lower your knees onto the floor. Uncurl your toes, keep your knees and feet hip width apart.

5   Breathe in. Sit back on your heels.

6   Breathe out. Lower your forehead to the floor and your elbows and lower arms.

7   Breathe in.

8   Breathe out. Slide your arms forward. Rest in comfort and ease.

9   Breathe in and out at least three times, until you are free of tension, specifically in the spine.

4

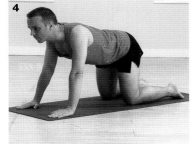

6

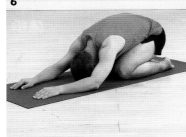

Benefits

- A restorative, calming pose.
- Stretches the arms and shoulders.
- Relaxes the spine and neck.
- Refreshes your mind and body.

Precautions

- Do not force your arms away from you, let them relax on to the floor, without any effort.

Modification

- If it is uncomfortable to place your forehead on the floor, make your hands into lightly-clenched fists; place one on top of each other.
- Rest your forehead onto your fists.
- Lengthen your spine, relax, and rest.

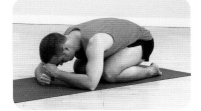

cat pose

Arching and stretching the spine like a cat. This posture really tones the abdominal area

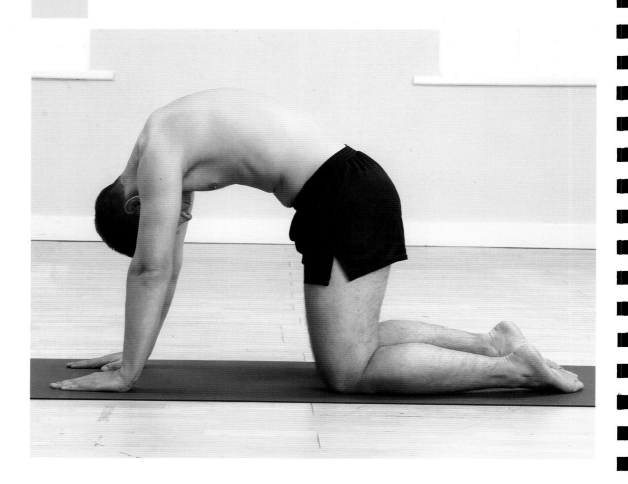

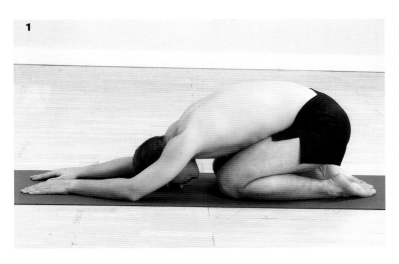

Method

1   Starting from Swan Pose.

2   Breathe in and out.

3   Breathe in. Look forward.

4   Breathe out. Come up onto all fours.

5   Breathe easy.

6   Position yourself with knees directly under your hips, shoulders, elbows, and wrists in line. Fingers should be lightly spread, elbows soft, drawn inwards. Draw your shoulders away from your ears. Lengthen your spine parallel to the floor, eyes to your navel.

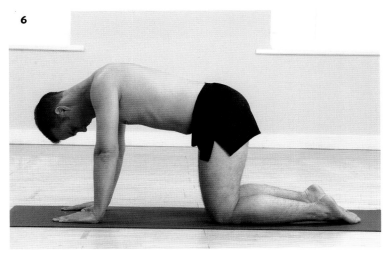

77

cat pose (continued)

7 Breathe in

8 Breathe out. Lower your chin towards your chest.

9 Draw your stomach inward and upward.

10 Arch your spine toward the ceiling, keeping your ears away from your shoulders. Look to your navel.

11 Breathe in. Slowly lower your spine.

12 Push your bottom upward and outward, slowly raise your eyes forward. Soften your face.

13 Breathe out. Lower your eyes. Let your spine relax and lengthen, parallel to the floor. Look to your navel. Let the top of your head relax toward the floor.

14 Breathe in and out.

15 Repeat four times.

16 Breathe normally.

■ *Remember, you are as young as the suppleness of your spine.*

10

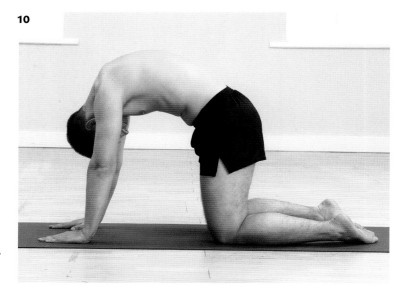

12

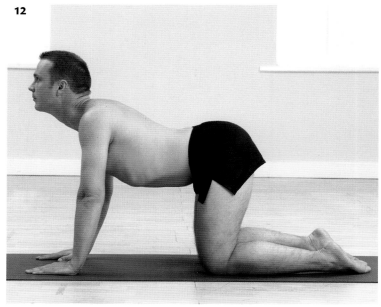

13

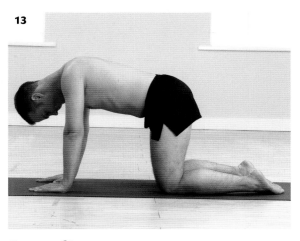

Benefits

- Firms the buttocks, stomach, thighs, and upper arms.
- Stretches and strengthens the spine and the neck.
- Encourages deep, rhythmic breathing.
- Creates a mindful awareness of breath and movement.
- Incorporates the pose and its contrapose in one fluid sequence.
- Softens the face and focuses the mind.

Precautions

- Draw your stomach in and up, do not pull it tight.
- Keep your shoulders away from your ears, do not hunch up.
- Do not force the chin on to your chest.
- Distribute your weight evenly, between your arms and legs.
- Do not let your spine collapse in the middle.
- Keep your toes stretched out, not curled up behind you.
- When your eyes and face are looking toward the ceiling, take care not to overstretch your neck, rather, lengthen your neck.

Modification
- If you suffer from arthritis or weakness in your hands and wrists; lightly clench your hands and support yourself this way.

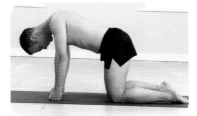

child pose

A restorative pose that strengthens the spinal and abdominal muscles.

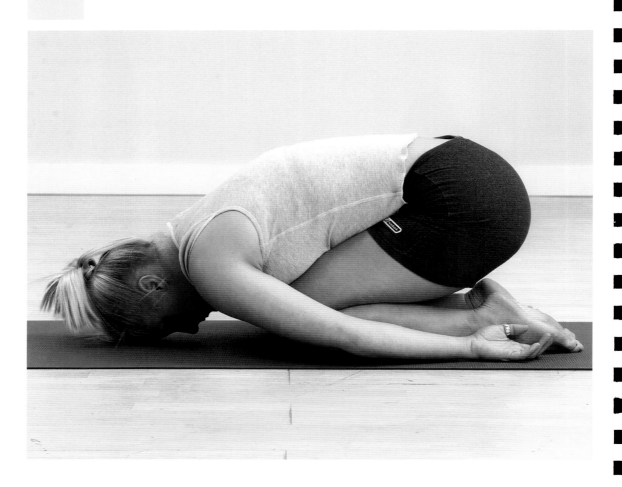

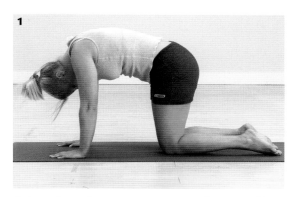

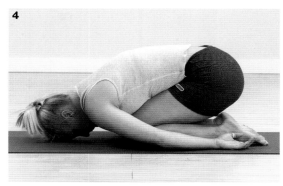

Method

1 Start from Cat Pose.
2 Breathe in and out.
3 Breathe in.
4 Breathe out. Sit back onto your heels. Place your forehead to the floor and arms to your sides. Palms facing the ceiling.
5 Breathe normally.
6 Rest, restore, rejuvenate.
7 Breathe into this pose until you are ready to continue your practice.

Benefits

• A restorative pose enabling you to let go, surrender, and relax.
• Enables us to tune into our breathing and alignment, recognizing the difference between tension and relaxation.
• Strengthens the spinal and abdominal muscles.
• Rejuvenates the mind, body, and spirit.

Precautions

• Keep your ears away from your shoulders.
• Wriggle and play around until you find the optimum posture for relaxation and rest.
• Allow the pose to restore your balance, rhythm, and vitality.
• Only come out of the pose when you are ready.
• Rest in this pose until your breath cues you into movement.

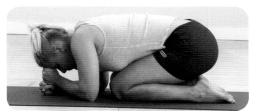

Modification
• Lightly clench the hands into fists.
• Place one fist on top of the other.
• Rest your forehead on your fists.
• Rest, restore, and rejuvenate.
• Stay in this pose until you are ready to continue.

seated pose (dandasana)

This is a preparation for the Seated Forward Bend. It also helps to tone and strengthen the abdominal area.

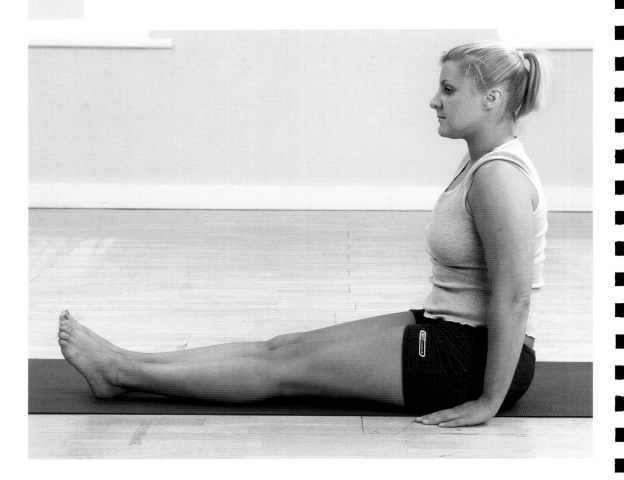

Method

1 Start from Child Pose.
2 Breathe in and out.
3 Breathe in. Sit on your heels.
4 Breathe out. Place your palms onto your thighs.
5 Breathe in. Place your left palm onto the floor, away from your hip.
6 Breathe out. Lean over to your left. Slide your buttocks onto the floor.
7 Breathe in. Stretch your legs out straight in front of you.
8 Breathe out. Make sure the backs of your legs touch the floor.
9 Breathe normally.
10 Position yourself with your legs, knees, and ankles together and your thighs rolling inward. Lift out your buttocks to sit on your sitting bones. Place your palms flat on the floor by the sides of your hips, fingers pointing toward your toes. Press your palms into the floor.
11 Lift up through your waist with your eyes forward and spine erect.
12 Breathe in.
13 Breathe out. Press the back of your thighs into the ground and the back of your heels into the floor. Extend your heels away from you. Draw your toes toward you. Keep your eyes forward and spine erect.
14 Breathe in and out three times. Listen to your breathing. When your breathing is smooth and rhythmic, you are ready for the Seated Forward Bend.
15 Breathe normally.

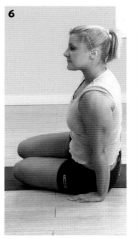
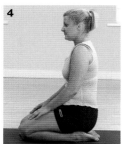
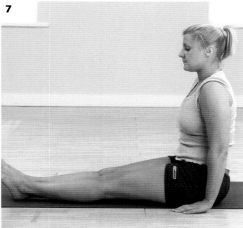
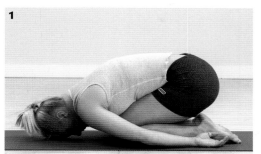

Benefits

- Reduces fat around the waist.
- Alleviates bloating sensations in the abdomen.
- Energy travels from your center, up through your spine, into your arms and hands and down through your legs, feet, and toes.
- Prepares the mind and body for the next poses.

Precautions

- Do not roll back into the base of your spine. Sit on your sitting bones.
- Spread your weight evenly along the width of your buttocks.
- Keep your face soft, do not strain or tense up.

Modification
- Place a folded blanket under your buttocks and lower spine to help support your spine in the upright position.
- Bend your elbows and knees.

seated forward bend 1 (paschimottanasana)

This initial version of the forward bend is a gentle stretch that slims and tones the entire back of the body.

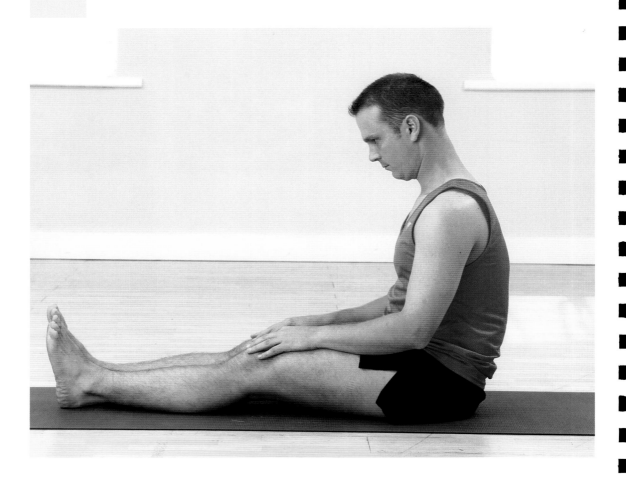

Method

1 Start from Seated Pose.

2 Breathe in and out.

3 Breathe in.

4 Breathe out. Place your palms onto your thighs, just above your knees.

5 Breathe in. Lift up through your waist.

6 Breathe out. Lower your chin toward your chest. Look at your toes.

7 Breathe in and out three times.

8 Breathe in. Look forward, raising your head and face.

9 Breathe out with your spine and neck erect and eyes forward.

Enjoy the feeling of calm this posture promotes.

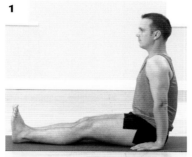

1

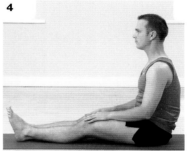

4

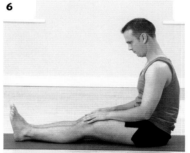

6

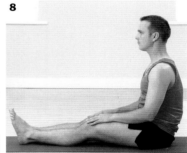

8

Benefits

- Forward Bends slim and tone all parts of the body, especially the arms, waist, abdomen, bottom, and legs.
- Strengthens the shoulders, back, and neck.
- Massages the internal organs, relieving constipation.
- Improves digestion.
- Releases tension in the spine.
- Aids concentration and invigorates the body and the mind.
- Develops perseverance and an awareness of how you feel, not how you look.

Precautions

- Don't hunch up. Keep your ears away from your shoulders.
- Roll your thighs inward and keep the backs of your legs on the floor.
- The backs of your heels should be away from you.
- Point your toes to the ceiling.
- For Seated Forward Bends 2 and 3 put your chest to your thighs, not your head to your knees.
- It is repetition and constant practice that lead to steady progress. Not pushing and pulling.

seated forward bend 2

Hands to thighs, extending the stretch.

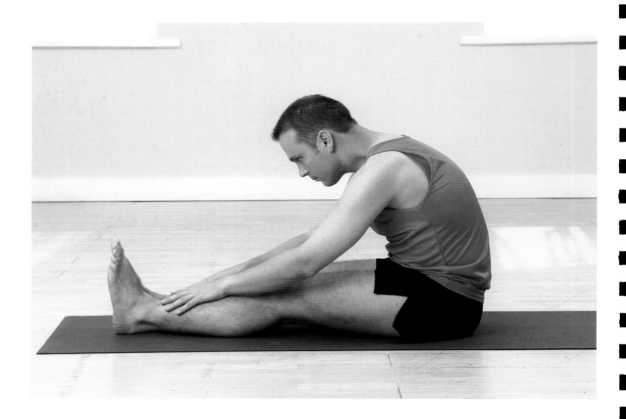

1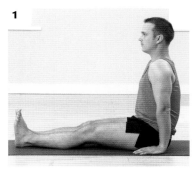

6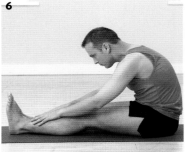

11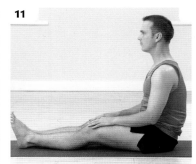

Method

1 Start from Seated Pose.

2 Breathe in and out.

3 Breathe in.

4 Breathe out. Place the palms of your hands onto your thighs.

5 Breathe in. Lift up through your waist.

6 Breathe out. Bend at your hips and fold forward. Reach out with your chest. Slide your hands down your legs with your elbows bent.

7 Breathe in. Look forward.

8 Breathe out. Lengthen your spine into the pose with your chest toward your thighs, ears away from your shoulders, eyes looking at your toes. Hold the pose.

9 Breathe in and out three times.

10 Breathe in. Look forward.

11 Breathe out. Come up to sitting. Slide your hands up your thighs with your eyes forward and spine erect.

12 Breathe normally.

■ *Congratulate yourself on your latest progress. Feel good!*

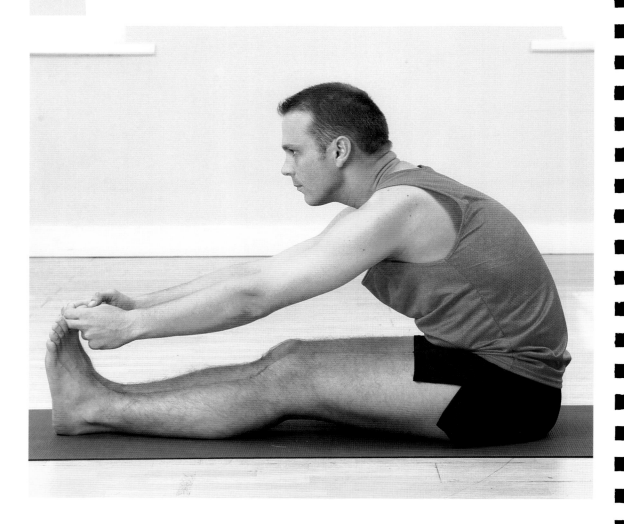

seated forward bend 3

Fingers hooked under your toes. Extending yourself further.

1

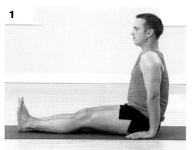

4

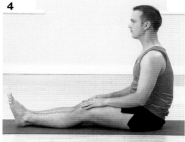

6

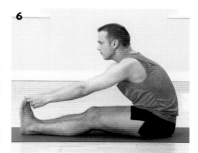

7

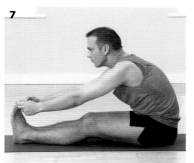

8

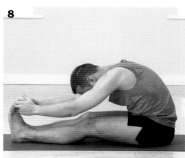

11

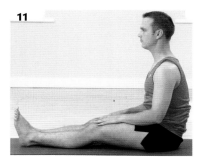

Method

1 Start from Seated Pose.

2 Breathe in and out.

3 Breathe in.

4 Breathe out. Place your palms onto your thighs.

5 Breathe in. Lift up through your waist.

6 Breathe out. Bend at your hips, fold forward. Hook your first two fingers behind each big toe.

7 Breathe in. Look forward.

8 Breathe out. Bend your elbows. Bring your chest toward your knees. Lengthen your spine. Hold the pose.

9 Breathe in and out three times.

10 Breathe in. Look forward, release your toes.

11 Breathe out. Come up to sitting. Slide your hands up your legs with your eyes forward and spine erect.

12 Breathe normally.

■ *Mental tensions dissolve as you surrender into the posture.*

fish pose (matsyasana)

The Fish Pose stretches the front of the body, opens your chest, and extends your spine.

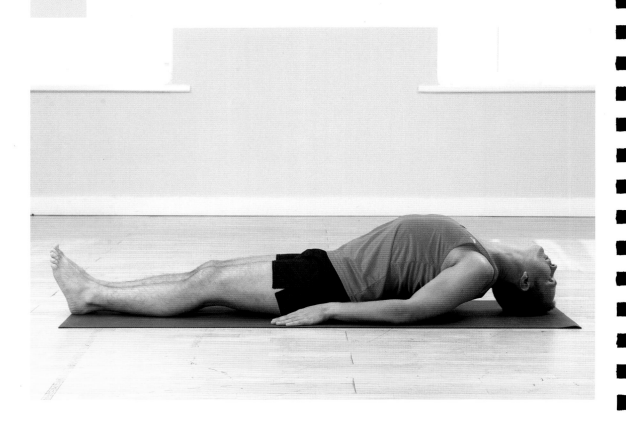

Method

1 Start from Seated Pose.

2 Breathe normally.

3 Roll yourself down onto the floor, so you are lying supine. Wriggle around until the length of your spine lies flat on the floor. Lift out your buttocks. Relax your spine onto the floor. Lower the back of your head to the floor. Let your chin relax toward your chest, with eyes looking directly toward the ceiling. Have your palms face up.

4 Breathe in and out.

5 Breathe in.

6 Breathe out. Bring your legs and feet together, with your arms by your sides and palms to the floor.

7 Breathe in. Gently arch your spine, raising your chest toward the ceiling, and ease the top of your head toward the floor.

8 Breathe out. Look behind you. Hold the pose.

9 Breathe in and out.

10 Breathe in. Arch your spine a little more.

11 Breathe out. Rest the top of your head on the floor, looking behind you. Now focus and hold the pose.

12 Breathe in and out three times.

13 Breathe in.

14 Breathe out. Lower your chest and push your head away. Sink your spine into the floor. Your eyes look to the ceiling.

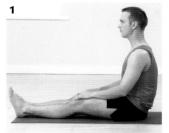
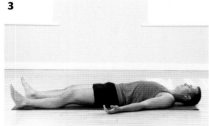
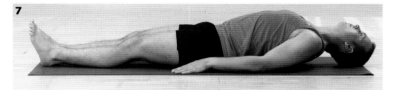
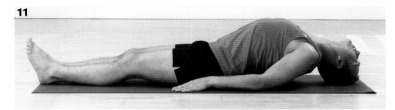
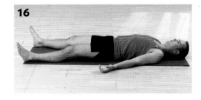

15 Breathe normally.

16 Lie on the floor in Relaxed Pose. Your legs and feet are apart, palms facing the ceiling, and eyes to the ceiling.

Benefits

- Firms and develops the chest.
- Increases strength and flexibility along the length of the spine.
- Stretches the neck and throat.
- Refreshes the face and head.

Precautions

- Be content to only raise the chest and arch the back a few inches.
- Do not rush. Feel your spine throughout the pose; be kind to your spine.

coil pose

This relaxing pose firms and slims the buttocks.

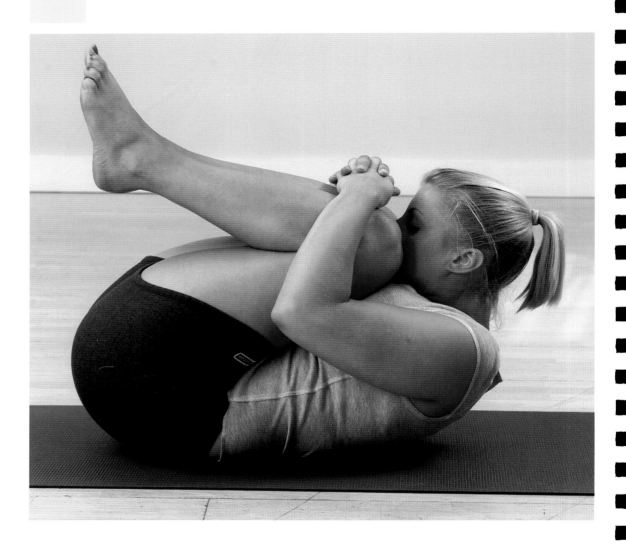

Method

1 Start from Relaxed Pose.

2 Breathe normally.

3 Bring your legs and feet together with arms to your sides, palms to the floor, eyes to the ceiling, and shoulders drawn away from your ears.

4 Breathe in.

5 Breathe out.
Bend your knees.

6 Bring them as close to your chest as you can.

7 Breathe in. Lace your fingers.

8 Place your hands over your knees.

9 Breathe out. Draw your knees and thighs toward your chest.

10 Breathe in. Raise your chin, nose, and eyes toward your knees.

11 Breathe out. Squeeze yourself into as small a ball as possible. Hold the pose.

12 Breathe in and out three times.

13 Breathe in.

14 Breathe out. Lower your head down onto the floor. Let your spine sink into the floor with your eyes looking at the ceiling. Your legs and feet are apart.

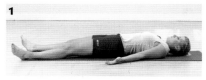

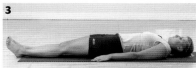

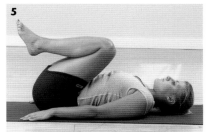

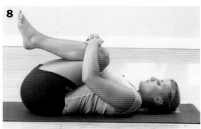

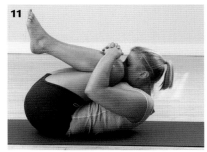

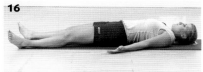

15 Breathe normally and learn to recognize the difference between tension and relaxation.

16 Rest in Relaxed Pose.

Benefits

- Slims and firms the buttocks and thighs.

- Increases strength and flexibility in the neck.

- Stretches the very top of the spine.

- Develops deep, rhythmic breathing.

Precautions

- If you have pain or problems with the neck area do not raise your head to your knees. Keep your head flat to the floor.

- Do not tense or strain.

Modification
- If you have neck problems, leave your head on the floor and follow breathing instructions. Concentrate on lengthening your spine along the floor.

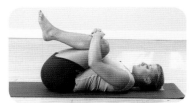

modified back bend/bridge pose (setu bandhasana)

Gives you an ageless, youthful body.

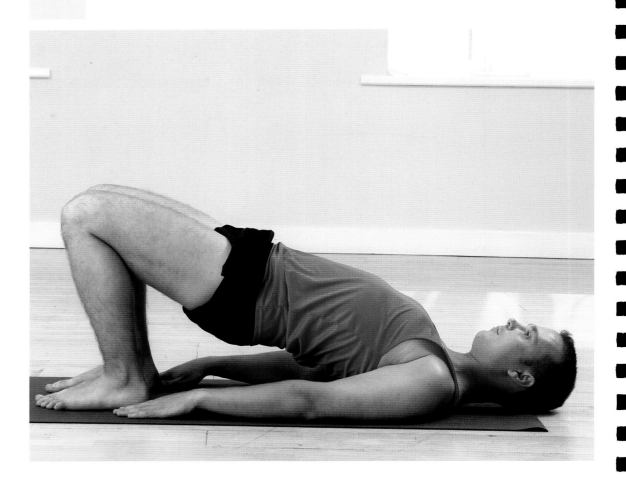

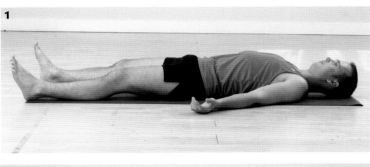

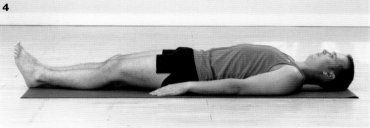

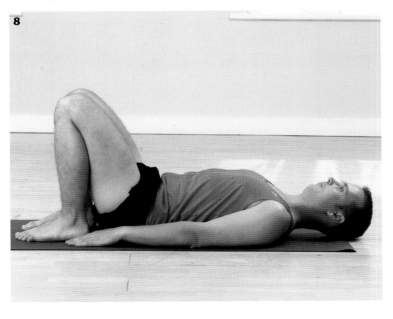

Method

1 Start from Relaxed Pose.

2 Breathe in and out.

3 Breathe in. Bring your legs and feet together.

4 Breathe out. Arms to your sides, palms facing the floor.

5 Breathe in. Lengthen your spine and neck.

6 Breathe out. Check the back of your head is resting on the floor, with your chin toward your chest and eyes to the sky.

7 Breathe in.

8 Breathe out. Bend your knees toward your chest. Place your feet onto the floor, hip width apart. Keep your heels close to your buttocks.

modified back bend/bridge pose (continued)

9 Breathe in. Push into the roots of your toes. Lift your bottom off the floor, raise it just a few inches.

10 Breathe out. Hold this position comfortably.

11 Breathe in. Raise your hips toward the ceiling, lifting your lower and middle spine off the floor. Keep your eyes to the ceiling.

12 Breathe out. Push into your feet to enable you to hold the pose with ease. Hold the pose.

13 Breathe in and out three times.

14 Breathe in.

15 Breathe out. Lower your spine and hips, rolling progressively back onto the floor.

16 Breathe in and out.

17 Repeat four times.

18 Breathe in.

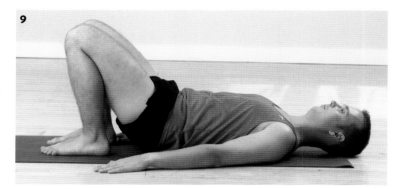

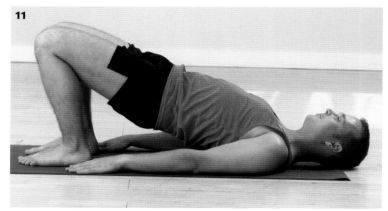

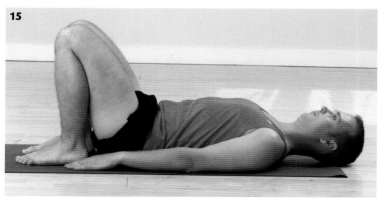

19

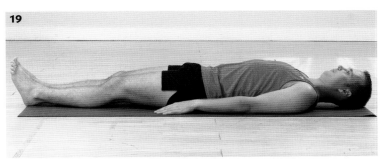

1 Prepare yourself for Modified Back Bend.
2 Lie on the floor, knees bent, feet flat.
3 Experiment with only lifting your bottom off the floor.
4 Learn to hold this posture in harmony with your breath.
5 Follow the instructions for Modified Back Bend to come out of the pose.

2

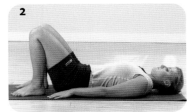

20

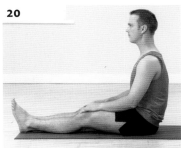

19 Breathe out. Push your feet away from you.

20 Breathe in. Immediately roll yourself up into Seated Pose.

21 Breathe out.

22 Breathe easy.

3

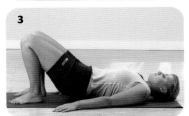

Benefits

- Gives the spine tremendous flexibility and strength.
- Strengthens and increases suppleness in the arms, wrists, and fingers.
- Relieves tension in the shoulders and lower back.
- Keeps the spine supple and youthful.

Precautions

- Do not let your hips drop toward the floor.
- Make sure your knees are hip width apart and your feet are parallel.
- Keep the back of your head to the floor.
- Do not raise your shoulders.
- Make sure your chest moves toward your chin.
- Your eyes should look directly to the ceiling.
- Always, always, practice the contrapose of Easy Forward Bend after this posture.

5

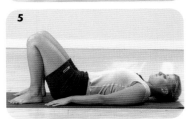

easy forward bend

The is the contrapose to the Bridge Pose. Arching your spine in the opposite direction.

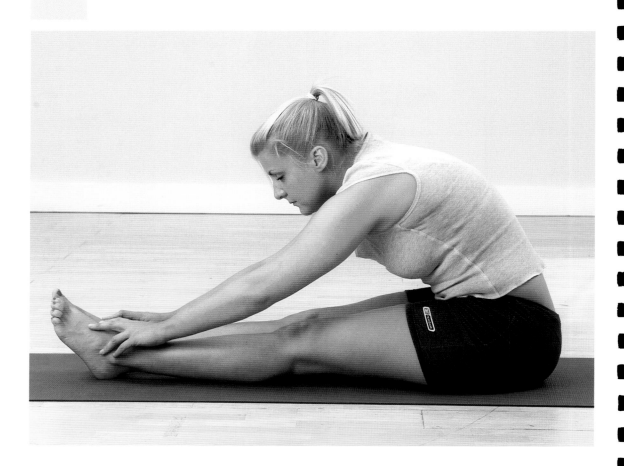

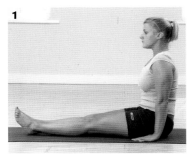

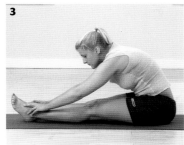

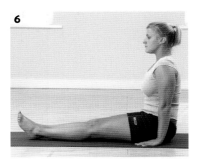

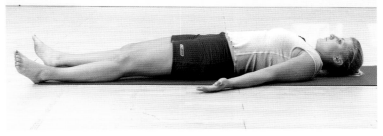

Method

1 Start from Seated Pose.

2 Breathe in.

3 Breathe out. Fold forward along the length of your legs. With no tension or forcing, move your chest toward your thighs. Your eyes should be looking at your lower legs. Roll your thighs inward. Hold the pose.

4 Breathe in and out three times.

5 Breathe in. Look forward.

6 Breathe out. Come up to sitting, with your eyes forward and spine erect.

7 Breathe in.

8 Breathe out. Roll down onto the floor. Your legs and feet are apart with your palms facing the ceiling, eyes to the ceiling also.

9 Breathe normally.

Benefits

- Allows your spine to arch in the opposite direction, releasing any tension in the spine or anxiety in the mind.
- Tones the abdominal area.
- Gently stretches the spine, hamstrings, and calves.
- Gives a feeling of rejuvenation and lightness.

Precautions

- There should be no tension in the spine and no tension in the body.
- Only go as far as you comfortably can, without strain or anxiety.

half shoulder stand (sarvangasana)

The Half Shoulder Stand revitalizes the whole system.

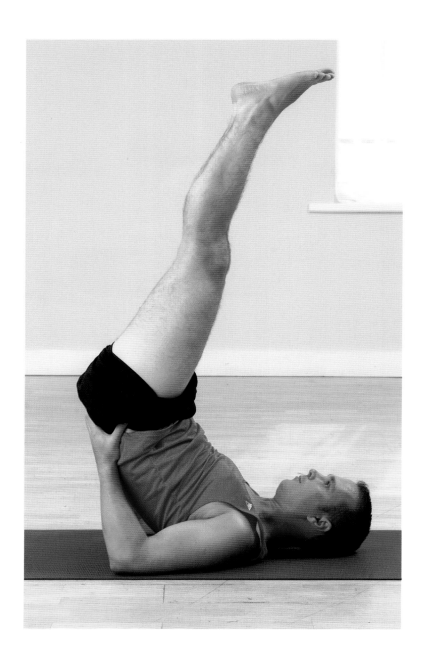

1

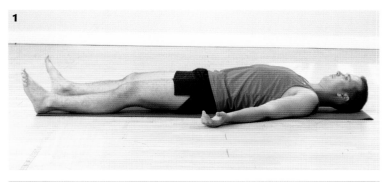

5

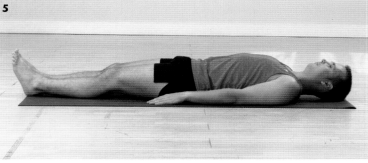

Method

1 Start from Relaxed Pose.

2 Breathe in and out.

3 Breathe in. Bring your legs and feet together.

4 Breathe out. Bring your arms to your sides.

5 Breathe in. Turn your palms to face the floor.

6 Breathe out. Lift your eyes to the ceiling, focus.

7 Breathe in.

8 Breathe out. Bend your knees toward your chest.

8

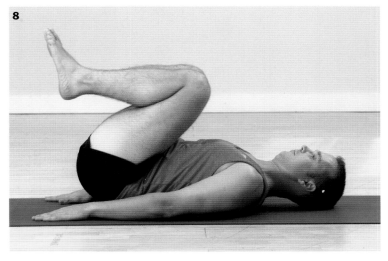

half shoulder stand (continued)

9 Breathe in.
   Raise your legs
   toward the ceiling.

10 Breathe out.
   Let your legs fall
   behind your
   head, lifting your
   bottom and lower
   spine off the floor.

11 Breathe in.
   Place your hands
   on your lower
   back, fingers
   pointing toward
   your buttocks,
   supporting
   your waist.

12 Breathe out.
   Raise your legs,
   toward the ceiling.
   Toes should be
   pointing upward.
   Support your
   weight by pressing
   along the length of
   your arms, from
   your shoulders
   to your elbows.

13 Breathe in and
   out three times.

14 Breathe in.

15 Breathe out. Bend
   your knees toward
   your face.

16 Breathe in. Place
   your palms flat
   on the floor.

9
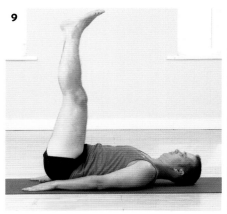

10
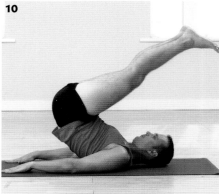

12
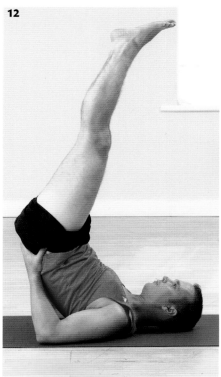

15
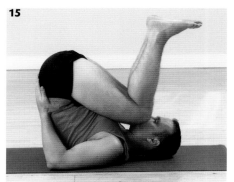

16
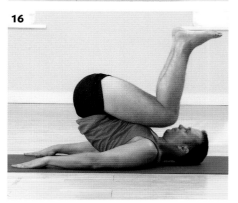

17

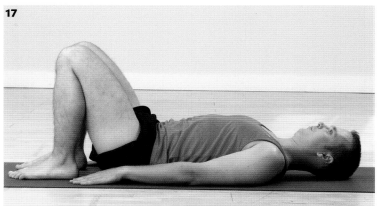

19

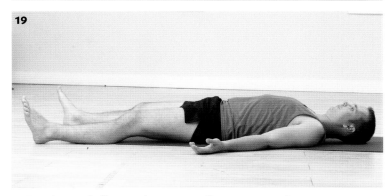

17 Breathe out. Roll your spine onto the floor. Keep your feet flat to the floor.

18 Breathe in.

19 Breathe out. Push your feet away from you. Your legs and feet should be apart, with your palms facing the ceiling.

20 Breathe normally.

Benefits

- Stimulates the flow of the blood to the face, skin and hair, revitalizing and rejuvenating.
- Tones and strengthens the buttocks, thighs, and backs of the legs.
- Slims and tones the abdomen.
- Strengthens the spine.
- Encourages deep abdominal breathing, massaging the lung and heart regions.
- This posture is excellent for the legs and can help prevent varicose veins, thread veins, and haemorrhoids.
- The thyroid gland is massaged, this can help stimulate a sluggish metabolism.
- Helps to ease insomnia and depression.

Precautions

- Do not practice this pose if you are pregnant, menstruating, have high blood pressure, head, or neck problems.
- Keep your legs together in the pose.
- Make sure your hands are evenly positioned.
- Focus and concentrate on your breath.

- Unless you have any of the contraindications, persevere with this pose. With practice you will gradually raise your bottom off the floor and raise your legs. It really is about perseverance.
- Try keeping your knees bent, and slowly, slowly learn to raise your legs (see Modification).

103

half shoulder stand (continued)

Modification

1 Prepare yourself for Half Shoulder Stand. Breathe in. Raise your legs to the ceiling. Keep your spine on the floor and eyes to the ceiling.

2 Breathe out.

3 Breathe in and out three times.

4 Breathe in. Breathe out. Bend your knees toward your chest.

5 Breathe in. Place your feet flat to the floor.

6. Breathe out. Push your feet away from you.

7 Breathe normally.

8 Rest in Relaxed Pose.

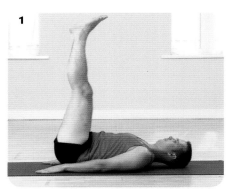

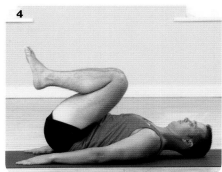

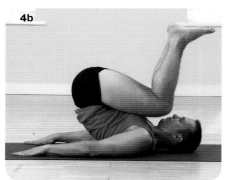

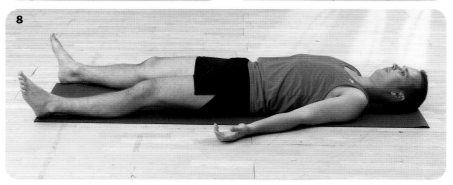

relaxed pose (savasana)

This is also known as Corpse Pose. The aim is to be completely still and to keep the mind empty from distracting thoughts.

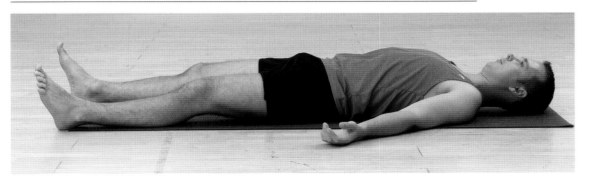

Method

1 Breathe normally.

2 Lie supine on the floor. Your legs and feet should be apart and your feet wider than your hips.

3 Keep your arms away from your sides and your palms facing the ceiling.

4 Wriggle around if necessary to ensure you have as much of your spine on the floor as possible.

5 Lift out your shoulders and buttocks.

6 Make sure you have the back of your head on the floor, not the top of your head.

7 Let your chin fall toward your chest and lift your eyes to the ceiling.

8 Lengthen your spine.

9 Imagine your spine sinking into the floor.

10 Close your eyes.

11 Each time you breathe out, imagine your spine sinking and relaxing into the floor.

12 Let yourself go. Surrender to your out breath.

13 Each time you breathe out, feel yourself letting go of any residual tensions or anxieties.

14 Rest in this pose for at least 3 breaths, with your body, mind, and breath as one.

Benefits

• Completely relaxes the body and mind.

• Eliminates fatigue, nervous tension, anxiety, depression, and irritability.

• Refreshes and revitalizes the whole body.

• This posture is often practiced between poses to ensure a proper flow of energy throughout the body and mind.

Precautions

• Take time to settle into this pose.

• Come out of the posture with mindful awareness.

• Your eyes should be closed to avoid distractions.

• If unwanted thoughts or distractions come into your mind, think of them as clouds on a summer's day, drifting across the horizon.

• Let them drift by, do not hold onto them.

Modification
• Place a blanket under the top of your shoulders and head.
• Keep your knees bent.
• Place a blanket under your knees.
• Make yourself as comfortable as possible.
• Experiment until you find the optimum pose, where you are in alignment, relaxed, and at ease.

cross-legged forward bend (sukhasana)

Part of a finishing sequence to prepare us for relaxation, concentration, and meditation.

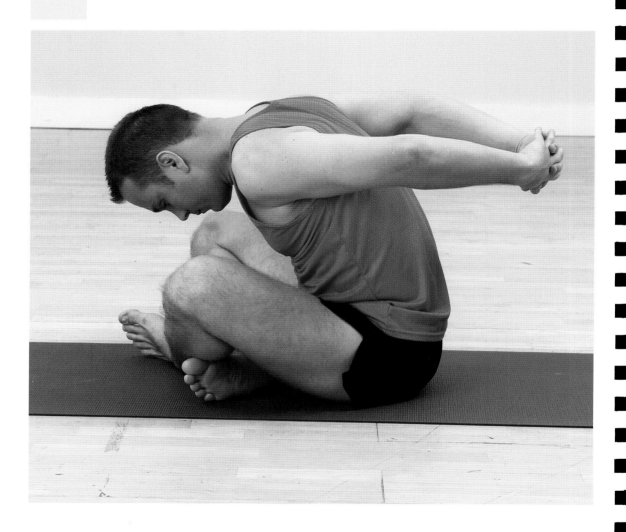

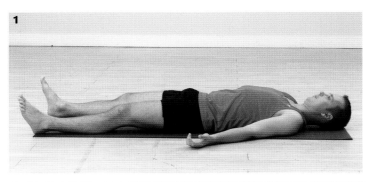

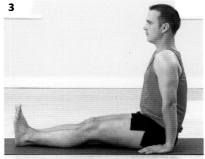

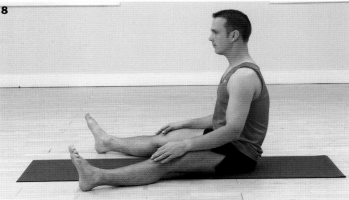

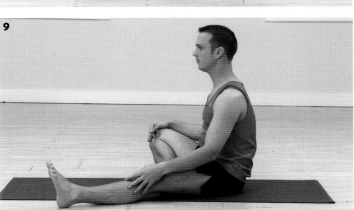

Method

1 Start from Relaxed Pose.
2 Breathe in and out.
3 Roll yourself up into Seated Pose.
4 Breathe in and out.
5 Breathe in. Sit with your spine erect and eyes forward.
6 Breathe out. Lift out your buttocks, so you are sitting comfortably.
7 Breathe in. Place your hands on the floor, either side of you.
8 Breathe out. Spread your legs apart.
9 Breathe in. Bend your right knee.
10 Breathe out. Place the heel of your right foot on the inside thigh of your left leg.

107

cross-legged forward bend (continued)

11 Breathe in. Bend your left knee.

12 Breathe out. Place the bottom of your left foot on your right shin.

13 Breathe in. Raise your arms to shoulder level.

14 Breathe out. Circle your arms behind you.

15 Breathe in. Lace your fingers.

16 Breathe out. Draw your hands away from you, opening your chest and shoulders.

17 Breathe in. Lift up through your waist.

18 Breathe out. Relax forward, aiming to rest your forehead on the floor. Look toward the floor. Your arms float up and eventually rise over your head.

19 Breathe in and out three times.

20 Breathe in. Look forward. Raise yourself up to a sitting position.

21 Breathe out. Lower your arms. Unlace your fingers, lower your arms to your side with palms to the floor.

22 Breathe normally.

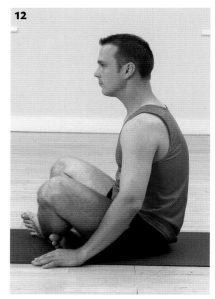

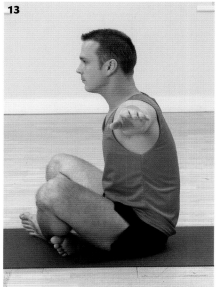

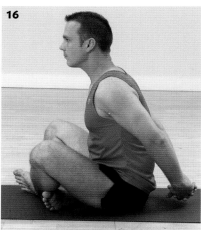

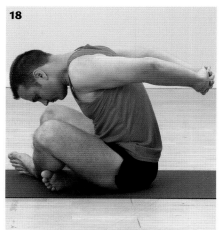

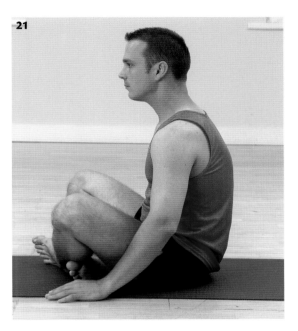

21

Modification
- Particularly if you have high blood pressure, before starting the pose place a support in front of you to rest your forehead on.
- To build up confidence in the pose, sit with your fingers laced behind you and work on drawing the arms away from you, do not go forward until you are ready.

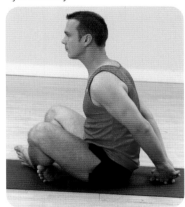

Benefits

- Massages and stimulates the abdominal area.
- Gives an intense stretch to the back and neck.
- Lengthens and strengthens the spine.
- Firms and tones the upper arms.
- Expands the chest.
- Tones and firms the breasts in women.
- Refreshes the mind and body.
- Promotes a feeling of peace and is calming and rejuvenating.

Precautions

- Do not clasp your hands together, your fingers should only be gently laced together.
- Do not raise your arms if it causes discomfort.
- At first you may find it difficult to place your forehead on the floor.
- You may feel like you are falling forward.
- Gently, slowly, find the place within yourself where you can hold the posture with grace and ease.
- If you have high blood pressure do not allow your head to fall lower than your heart.

cross-legged backward bend (sukhasana)

This is a contrapose to Lotus Forward Bend, where you arch your spine in the opposite direction.

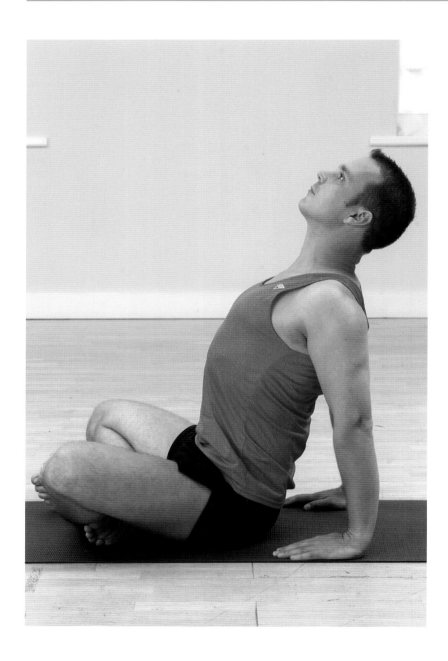

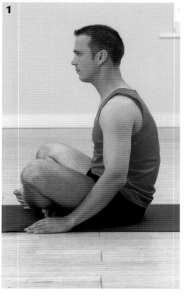

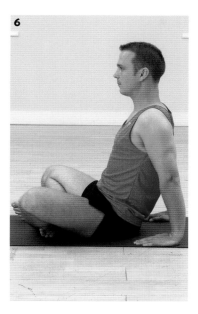

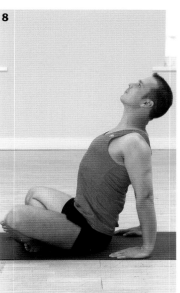

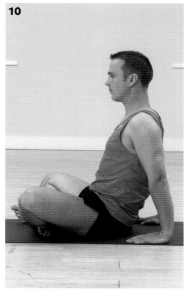

Method

1 Start in a seated position with your legs crossed.

2 Breathe in and out.

3 Breathe in.

4 Breathe out. Place your palms on the floor either side of your hips. Your fingers should be pointing toward your toes.

5 Breathe in.

6 Breathe out. Slide your hands behind you. The tips of your fingers should be in line with your hips.

7 Breathe in. Gently arch your spine, raising your chest to the ceiling.

8 Breathe out. Look up to the ceiling. Hold the pose. Push into your hands to support yourself.

9 Breathe in and out three times.

10 Breathe in. Look forward. Lower your chest.

cross-legged backward bend (continued)

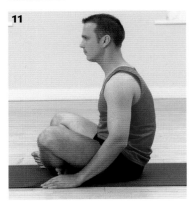

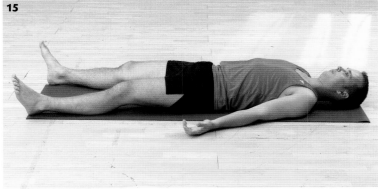

11 Breathe out. Come up to sitting position with your eyes forward and spine erect.

12 Breathe normally.

13 Stretch your legs out in front of you.

14 Roll down onto the floor.

15 Rest in Relaxed Pose.

Benefits

- Tones and stretches the abdominal area.
- Stretches and strengthens the back.
- Can help ease backache.
- Tones the chest.
- Produces a feeling of calm and peace.

Precautions

- Do not collapse your spine as you raise your chest.
- Your elbows should be rolled in. Keep them soft, not locked.

Modification
- If this posture is too difficult, just sit comfortably in a cross-legged position and listen to your breathing.

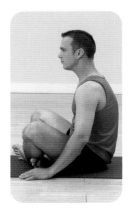

concentration pose

1

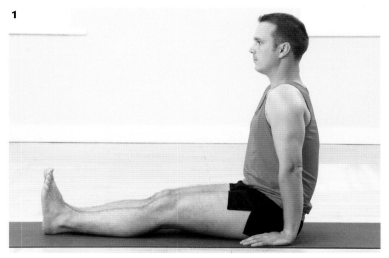

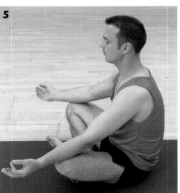

13

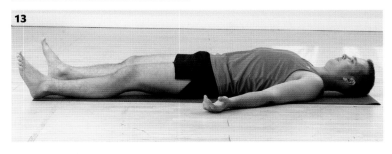

Method

1 Start from Seated Pose.
2 Breathe in and out.
3 Breathe in. Make your thumb and first finger of each hand touch.
4 Breathe out. Point three fingers outward from your hands.
5 Breathe in. Rest the back of your arms on your knees. Close your eyes and imagine they are looking to the middle of your forehead.
6 Breathe out. Sit in comfort. Take five good, deep breaths in and out.
7 Breathe calmly. Listen to your breathing.
8 Be aware of how much deeper, smoother, and more rhythmic your breathing has become.
9 Rest comfortably in this pose.
10 Breath with mind and body united, at peace.
11 Stay in this pose until you are ready to lie on the floor for relaxation.
12 When you are ready, lower your eyes, stretch your legs out in front of you, and roll yourself down onto the floor. Move your legs and feet apart, arms away from your sides.
13 Rest in Relaxed Pose.

Benefits

• This posture teaches us to sit comfortably, without distraction, so we may meditate in peace.

113

curl up, roll up, sit up

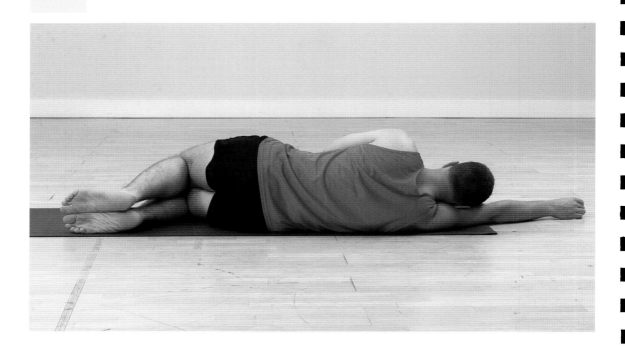

Method

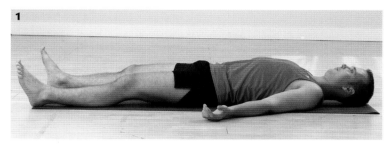

1. Start from Relaxed Pose.
2. Breathe calmly.
3. Bring your legs and feet together, arms to your sides, and palms to the floor.
4. Breathe in. Raise your arms above your head, the back of your hands facing the floor. Have a really good stretch, toes to fingertips.
5. Breathe out.
6. Breathe in.
7. Breathe out. Lower your left arm to your left side.
8. Breathe in. Roll over onto your right-hand side.
9. Breathe out. Bend your knees. Your left hand should be resting either on the floor or on your hip, your head resting in the crook of your right arm.
10. Breathe in and out three times.
11. Breathe in. Roll up to sitting.
12. Breathe out. Sit in an easy, cross-legged posture in comfort.
13. Breathe calmly.

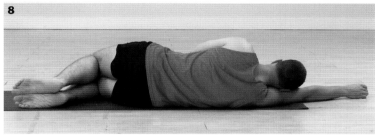

Benefits

- These movements gently ease us out of relaxation, increasing the circulation and that feelgood factor.

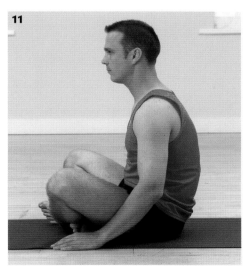

hands to eyes/hair tugs/stroke face

Increases the circulation of the blood to the face and head.

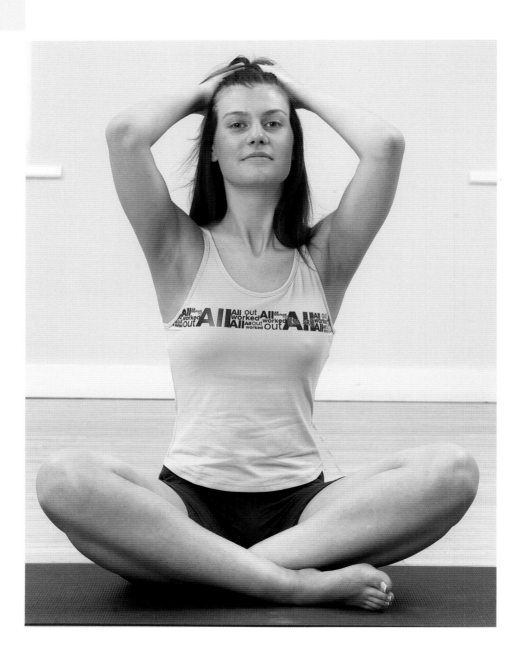

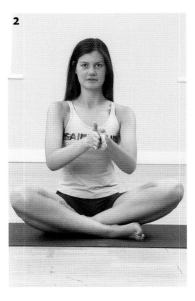

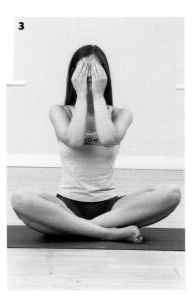

Method

1 Start from Seated Pose, legs crossed.

2 Breathe in. Briskly rub the palms of your hands together.

3 Breathe out. Place your palms over your closed eyes.

4 Breathe in. Open your fingers.

5 Breathe out. Open your eyes.

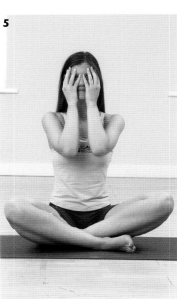

hands to eyes/hair tugs/stroke face (continued)

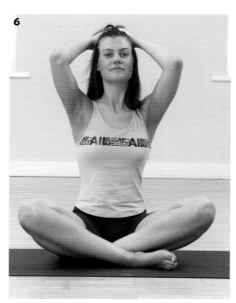

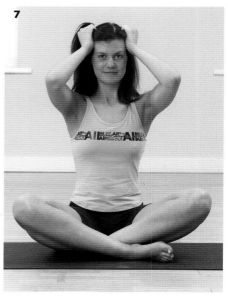

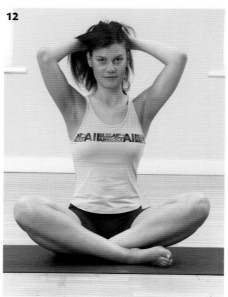

6 Breathe in. Push your fingers into your scalp.

7 Breathe out. Grab hold of as much hair as you can.

8 Breathe calmly.

9 Gently tug your hair, up and away from your scalp six times.

10 Then tug your hair downward six times.

11 Breathe in. Push your fingers into the nape of your neck.

12 Breathe out. Grab as much hair as you can.

13 Breathe calmly.

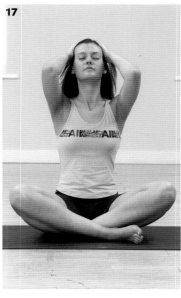

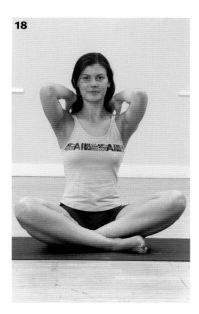

Benefits

- Can help disperse the fleshy deposit that develops under the chin
- Promotes healthy, strong shining hair
- Stimulates the flow of the blood into the scalp and hair follicles to maintain the scalp and hair in good condition.
- Wakes us up and revitalizes.

Precautions

- Do not overdo the tugging part or you may inadvertently pull your hair out!

14 Try six tugs upward.

15 Now try six tugs downward.

16 Breathe calmly.

17 With open palms, starting just below your chin, stroke your face, and the top of your head.

18 Stroke the back of your head, the nape of your neck, and across your shoulders.

19 Shake out your hands.

20 Repeat three times.

21 Breathe calmly.

Modification
- For those whose hair is receding, or who have very short or no hair, keep your fingers gently pushing into the scalp. Push upward and downward.

stand up

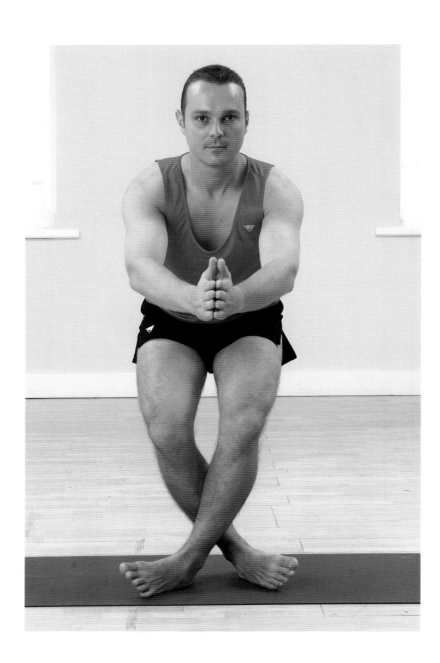

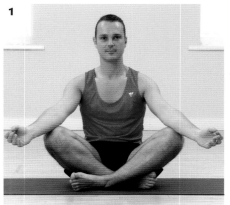

1

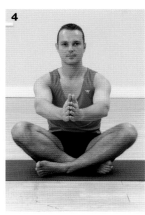

4

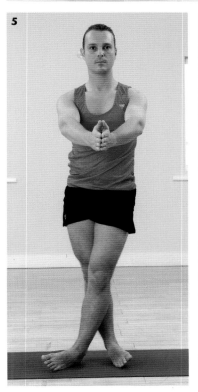

5

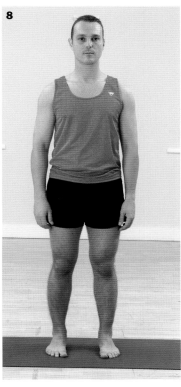

8

Method

1 Start in a cross-legged, seated position.
2 Breathe in and out.
3 Breathe in. Raise your arms out to the side to shoulder level.
4 Breathe out. Place your palms together.
5 Breathe in. With your eyes forward, lift up through your waist. Come up to standing.
6 Breathe out. Lower your arms to your sides. Uncross your feet.
7 Breathe in. Walk your feet to hip width apart.
8 Breathe out. Stand in Mountain Pose. Keep your eyes forward and spine erect. Keep your breathing deep, smooth, and rhythmic.

Benefits

- Strengthens the abdomen and legs.
- Improves balance and makes you feel great.

Precautions

- This posture takes time and technique to achieve.
- Persevere, you will be amazed how good you feel when you master the pose.

stand up (continued)

Modification

1 Start from a cross-legged, seated position.

2 Stretch your legs out in front of you.

3 Place your left hand to the floor away from your side.

4 Roll over onto your left buttock.

5 Curl your legs beneath you.

6 Roll onto your knees so you are kneeling on the floor.

7 Place your right foot flat on the floor in front of you.

8 Place your left foot parallel to your right foot.

9 Come up to standing.

10 Stand in Mountain Pose.

11 Breathe calmly.

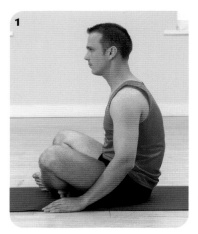

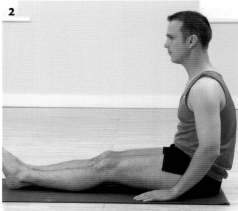

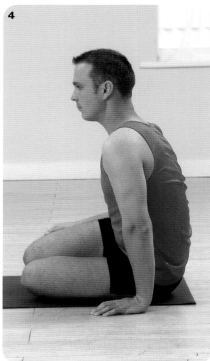

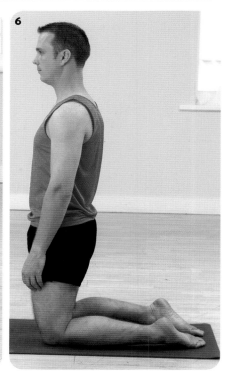

7

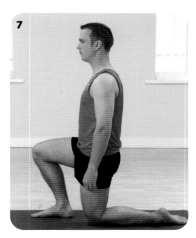

9

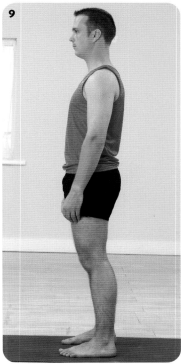

10

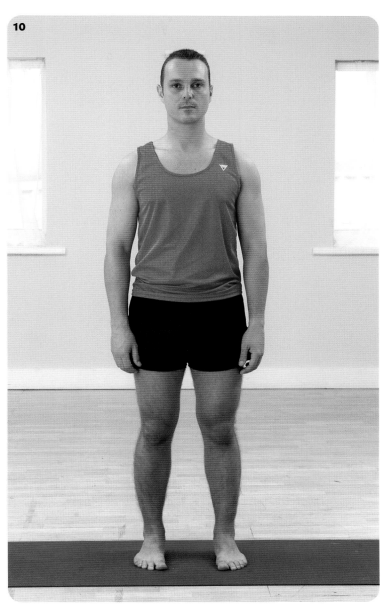

closing breath

This posture helps to finish the sequence by closing down the energy centers.

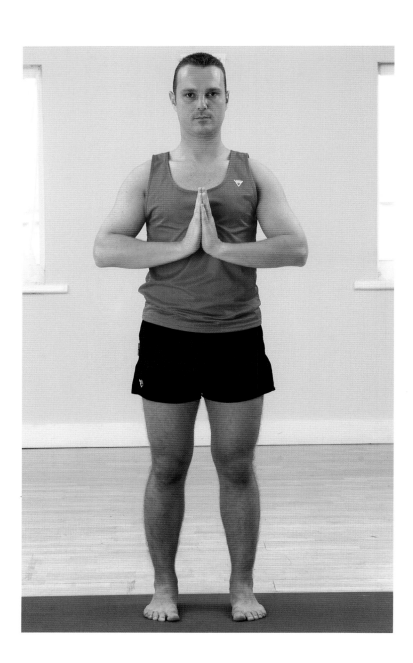

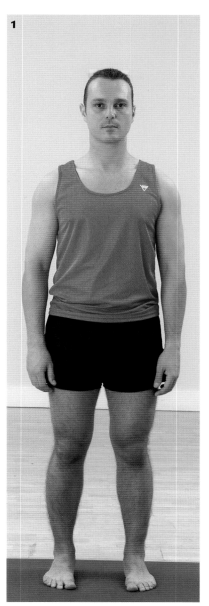

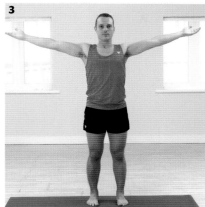

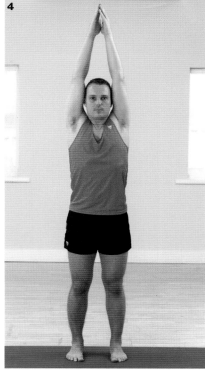

Method

1 Start from Mountain Pose.

2 Breathe in and out.

3 Breathe in. Raise your arms above your head. Arms straight, elbows soft.

4 Place your palms together above your head.

closing breath (continued)

5 Breathe out. Lower your palms to your chest.

6 Then move your arms to your sides.

7 Breathe in. Raise your arms above your head. Palms together.

8 Breathe out. Lower your palms to your chest, breathing out with a big sigh.

9 Move your arms to your sides.

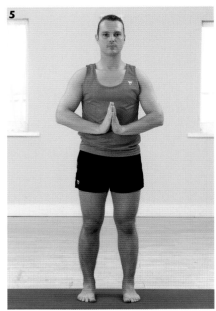

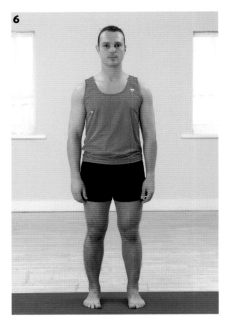

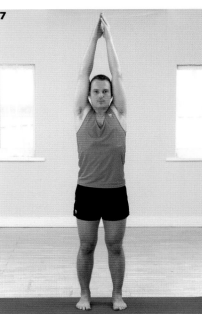

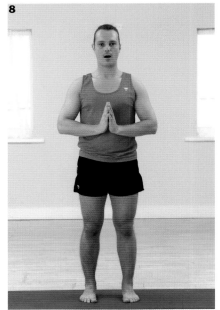

9

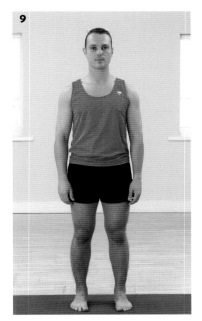

11

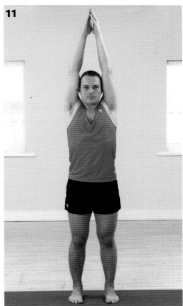

12

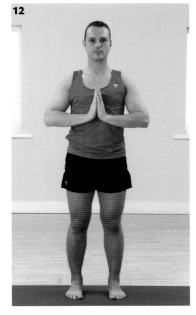

10 Breathe in. Raise your arms above your head.

11 Place your palms together.

12 Breathe out. Lower your palms to your chest.

13 Breathe in. Bring your feet together.

14 Breathe out. Look forward, take a small bow.

15 Breathe in. Take your feet back to hip width apart.

16 Breathe out. Bring your arms to your sides and keep your eyes forward. Keep your spine erect.

17 Stand in Mountain Pose.

18 Breathe calmly.

Benefits

- Closes down the energy centers. Energy is within us, stored for when we need it.

- Gives a feeling of closure to the sequence.

- Creates a feeling of calm and well-being.

Precautions

- Do not overstretch.

- Keep your focus and don't rush.

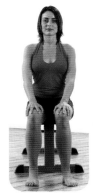

Modification
- May be practiced sitting on an armless chair. or lying supine on the floor.

127

Yoga 20-Minute Sequences

7-a-day, every day

Read the instructions carefully, until you are familiar with them. Start with the introductory sequence, 7-a-Day, Every Day. When this becomes easy, and you are familiar with the techniques, move on to Sequence 1.

A good idea is to look at the sequence the night before. Read the instructions, follow the breathing pattern, and imagine yourself practicing the pose. Or, practice with a friend and take it in turns to read the postures out loud while the other practices.

When Sequence 1 becomes easy, move onto Sequence 2 then 3, and so on.

Never rush. If you are running out of time, it is better to do less, practicing with grace and ease, than to finish the sequence at all costs and end up feeling stressed.

Include Deep Relaxation, Concentration, and Meditation whenever you have more time. Or, choose to practice each technique by itself for twenty minutes, whenever you feel the need. Ideally, you would set aside a time each day, purely for meditation practice.

Always finish any sequence or personal practice plan with the Mountain Pose and the Closing Breath.

Standing in Mountain Pose after practice, allows the breathing to return to normal. It enables the body and mind to experience the benefits of the poses and gives a feeling of being grounded and centered.

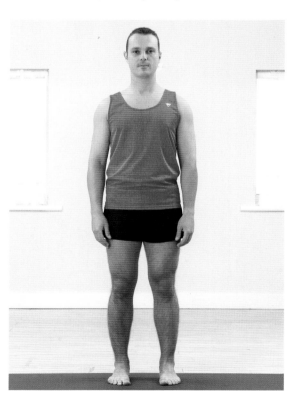

1. Mountain Pose (4 breaths)

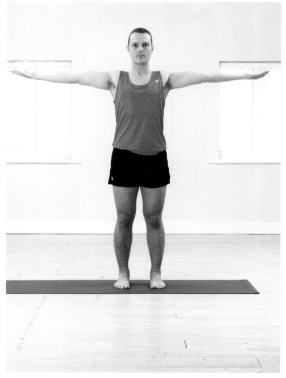

2. Complete Breath (x3)

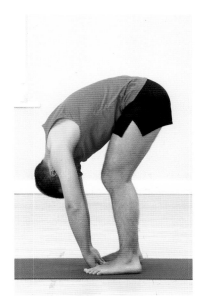

3. Refresher Breath (x3)

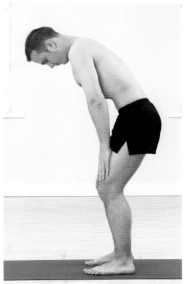

4. Abdominal Lift (x1)

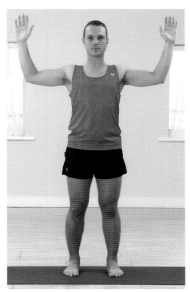

5. Sun Salutation (x1)

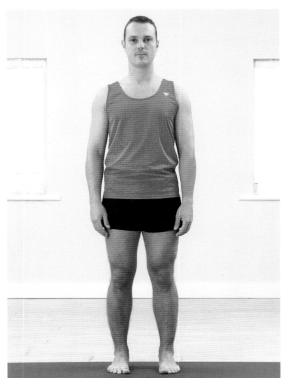

6. Mountain Pose (x4)

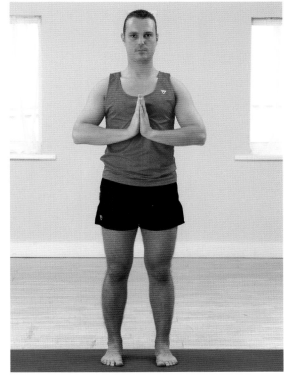

7. Closing Breath

sequence 1

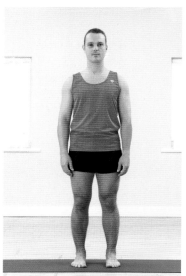

1 Mountain Pose (4 breaths)

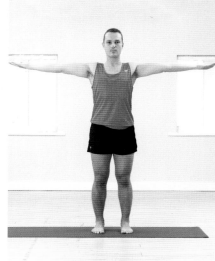

2 Complete Breath (x1)

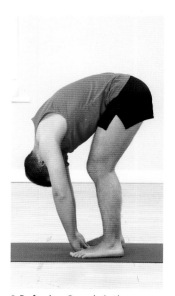

3 Refresher Breath (x1)

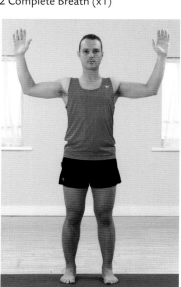

4 Abdominal Lift (x1)

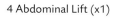

5 Sun Salutation (x1)

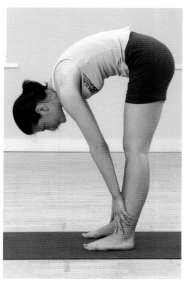

6 Standing Forward Bend 1 (x2)

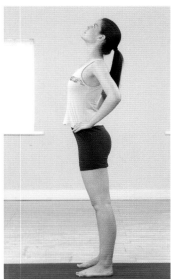

7 Standing Back Bend (x1)

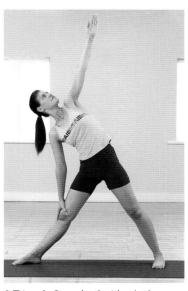

8 Triangle Pose, both sides (x1)

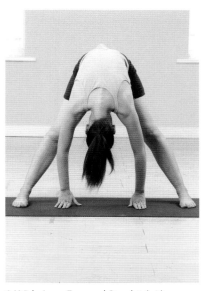

9 Wide Legs Forward Bend 1 (x2)

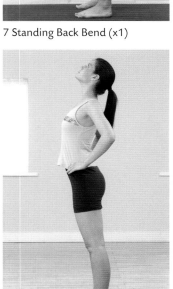

10 Standing Back Bend (x1)

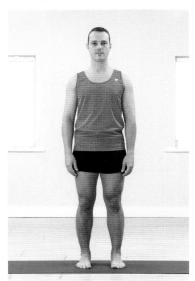

11 Mountain Pose (4 breaths)

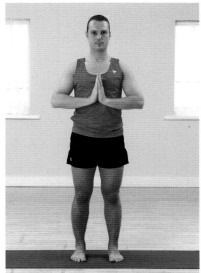

12 Closing Breath

sequence 2

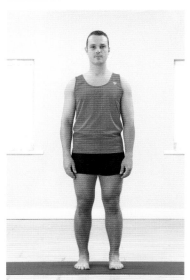

1 Mountain Pose (4 breaths)

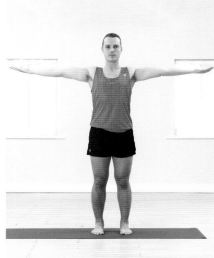

2 Complete Breath (x1)

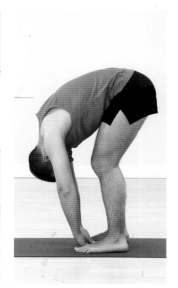

3 Refresher Breath (x1)

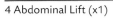

4 Abdominal Lift (x1)

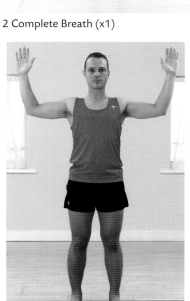

5 Sun Salutation (x1)

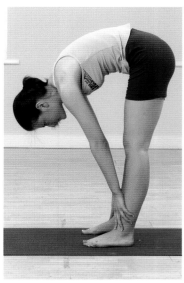

6 Standing Forward Bend 1 (x2)

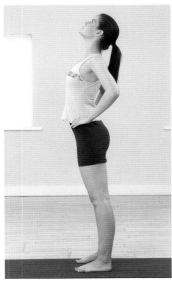 

7 Standing Back Bend (x1)

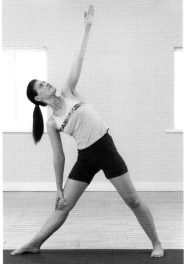

8 Triangle Pose, both sides (x1)

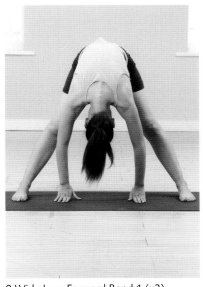

9 Wide Legs Forward Bend 1 (x2)

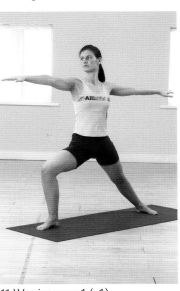 

10 Standing Back Bend (x1)

11 Warrior, pose 1 (x1)

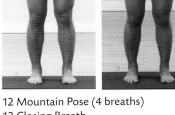

12 Mountain Pose (4 breaths)
13 Closing Breath

sequence 3

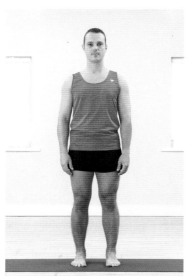

1 Mountain Pose (4 breaths)

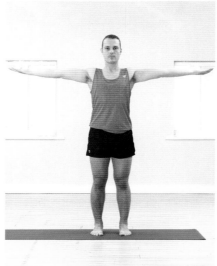

2 Complete Breath (x1)

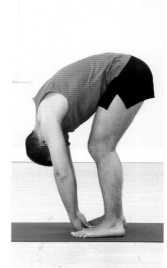

3 Refresher Breath (x1)

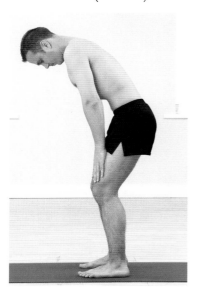

4 Abdominal Lift (x1)

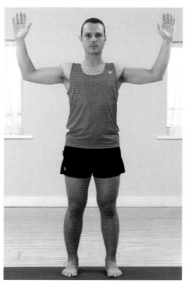

5 Sun Salutation (x1)

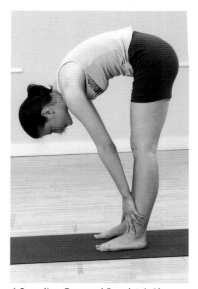

6 Standing Forward Bend 1 (x2)

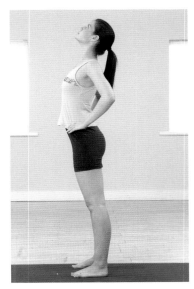

7 Standing Backward Bend (x1)

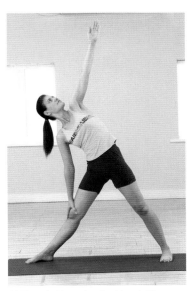

8 Triangle Pose, both sides (x1)

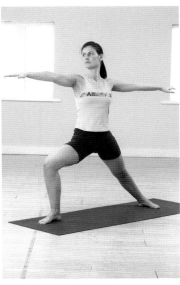

9 Warrior, pose 1 (x1)

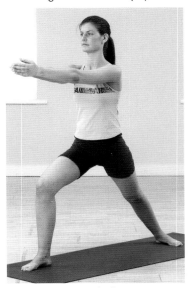

10 Warrior, pose 2 (x1)

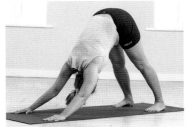

11 Downward Dog (x1)

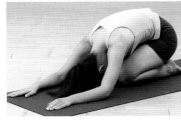

12 Swan (x1)

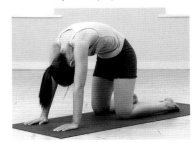

13 Cat Pose (x1)

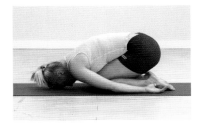

14 Child Pose (x1)

sequence 3 (continued)

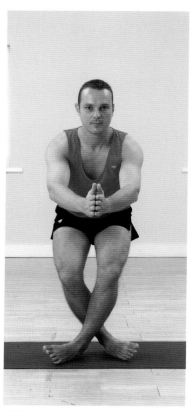

15 Stand Up (x1)

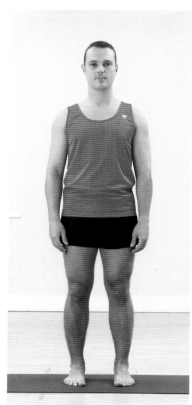

16 Mountain Pose (4 Breaths)

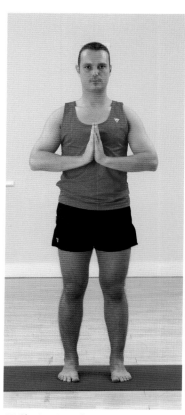

17 Closing Breath

sequence 4

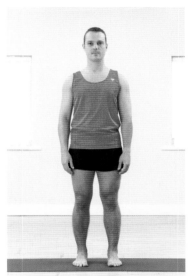

1 Mountain Pose (4 breaths)

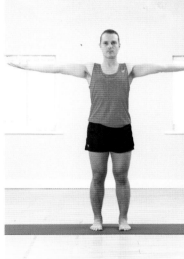

2 Complete Breath (x1)

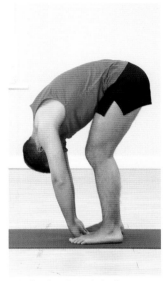

3 Refresher Breath (x1)

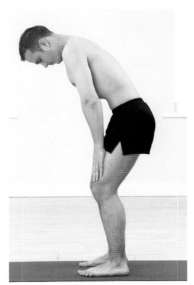

4 Abdominal Lift (x1)

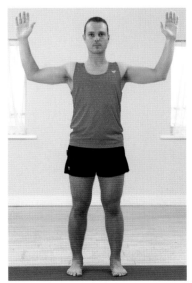

5 Sun Salutation (x1)

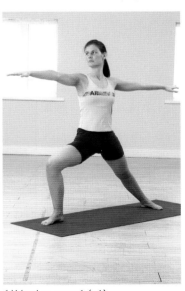

6 Warrior, pose 1 (x1)

sequence 4 (continued)

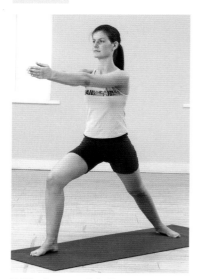

7 Warrior, pose 2 (x1)

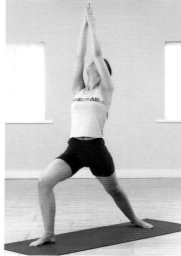

8 Warrior, pose 3 (x1)

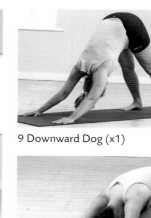

9 Downward Dog (x1)

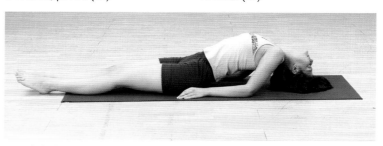

10 Swan (x1)

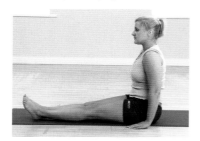

11 Seated Pose (4 breaths)

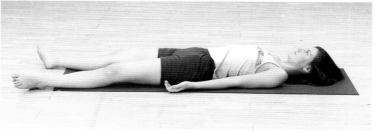

13 Fish (x1)

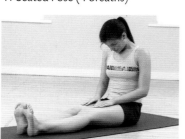

12 Seated Forward Bend 1 (x1)

14 Relaxed Pose (4 breaths)

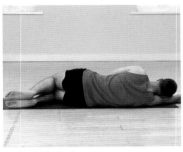

15 Curl Up (x1)

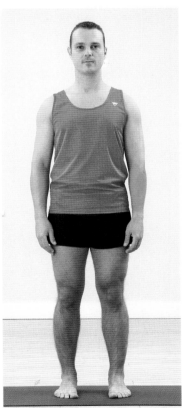

16 Sit Up (x1)

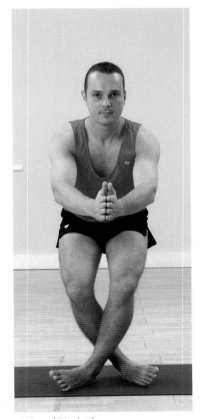

17 Stand Up (x1)

18 Mountain Pose (4 breaths)

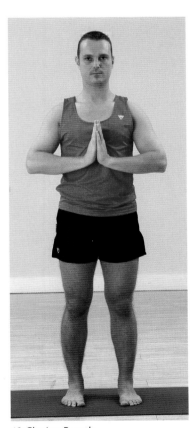

19 Closing Breath

sequence 5

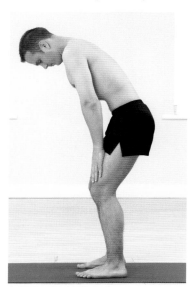

1 Mountain Pose (4 breaths)

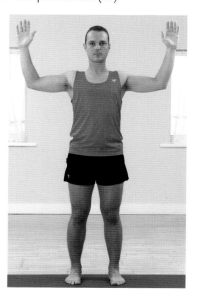

2 Complete Breath (x1)

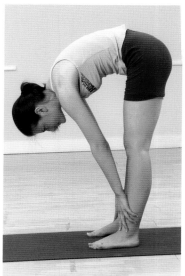

3 Refresher Breath (x1)

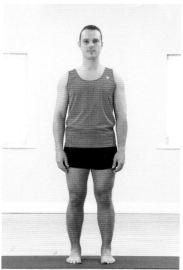

4 Abdominal Lift (x1)

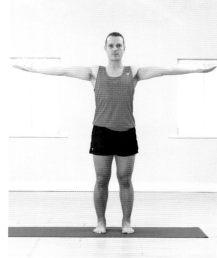

5 Sun Salutation (x1)

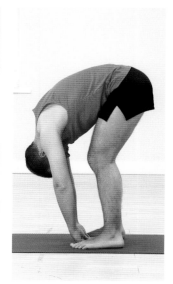

6 Standing Forward Bend 1 (x2)

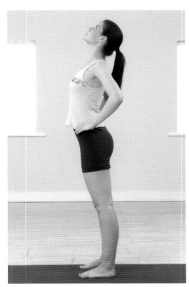

7 Standing Backward Bend (x1)

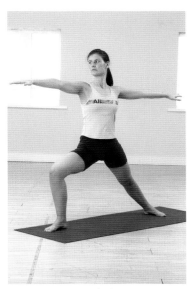

8 Warrior, pose 1 (x1)

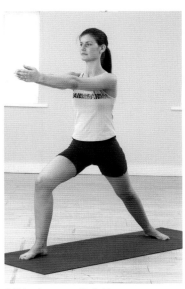

9 Warrior, pose 2 (x1)

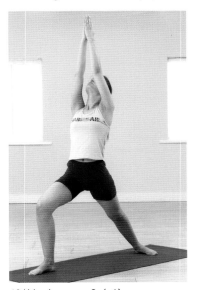

10 Warrior, pose 3 (x1)

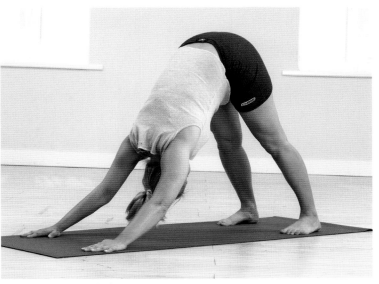

11 Downward Dog (x1)

sequence 5 (continued)

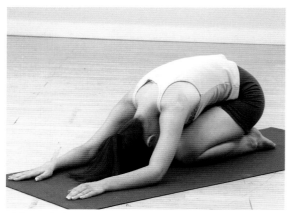

12 Swan (x1)

13 Seated Pose (4 breaths)

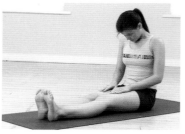

14 Seated Forward Bend 1 (x1)

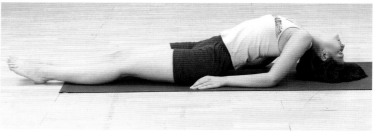

15 Fish (x1)

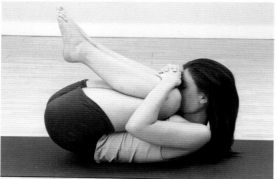

16 Coil (x1)

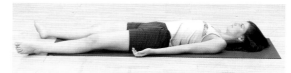

17 Relaxed Pose (4 breaths)

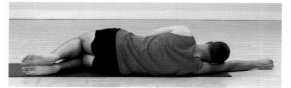

18 Curl Up (x1)

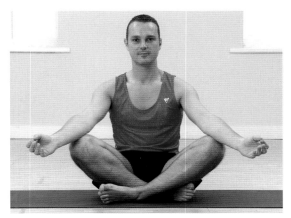

19 Sit Up (x1)

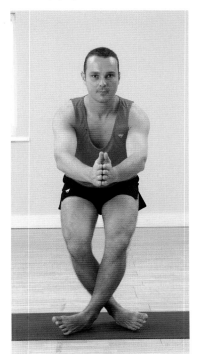

20 Stand Up (x1)

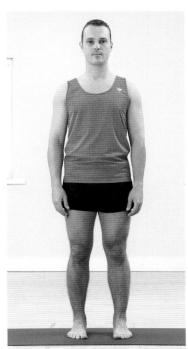

21 Mountain Pose (4 breaths)

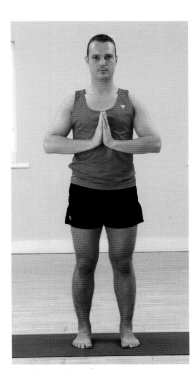

22 Closing Breath

sequence 6

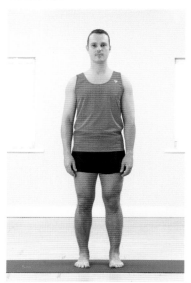

1 Mountain Pose (4 breaths)

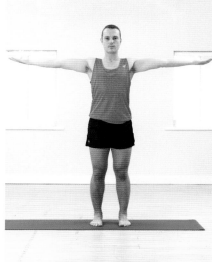

2 Complete Breath (x1)

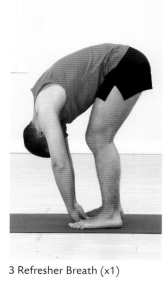

3 Refresher Breath (x1)

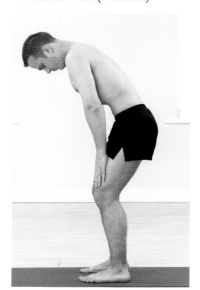

4 Abdominal Lift (x1)

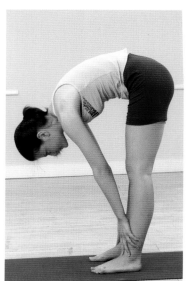

5 Standing Forward Bend 1 (x1)

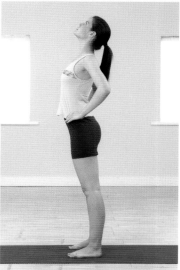

6 Standing Backward Bend (x1)

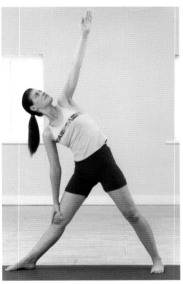

7 Triangle Pose, both sides (x1)

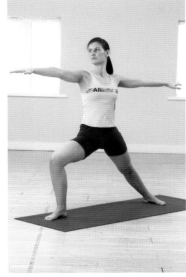

8 Warrior, pose 1 (x1)

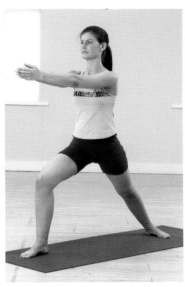

9 Warrior, pose 2 (x1)

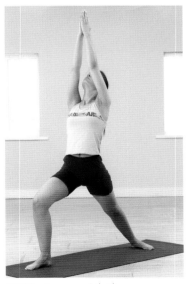

10 Warrior, pose 3 (x1)

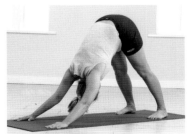

11 Downward Dog (x1)

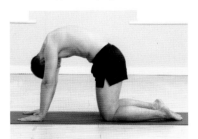

13 Cat Pose (x1)

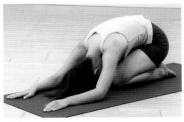

12 Swan (x1)

sequence 6 (continued)

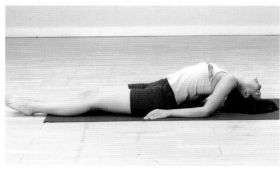

14 Fish Pose (x1)

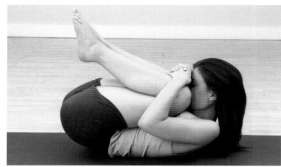

15 Coil (x1)

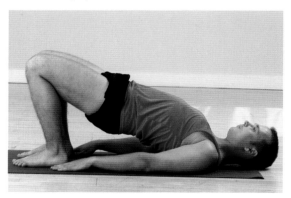

16 Modified Back Bend (x1)

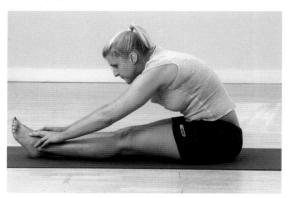

17 Easy Forward Bend (x1)

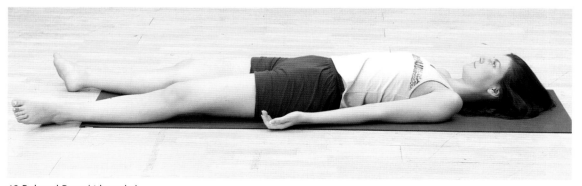

18 Relaxed Pose (4 breaths)

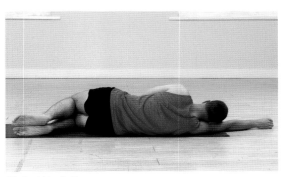

19 Curl Up (x1)

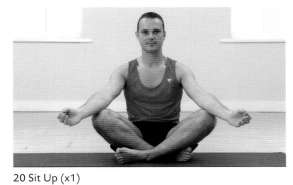

20 Sit Up (x1)

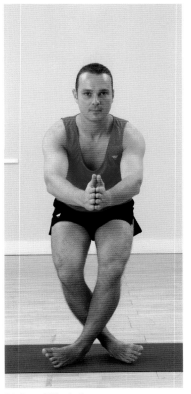

21 Stand Up (x1)

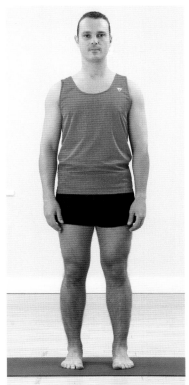

22 Mountain Pose (4 breaths)

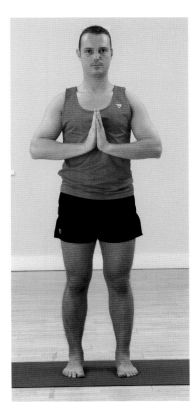

23 Complete Breath

sequence 7

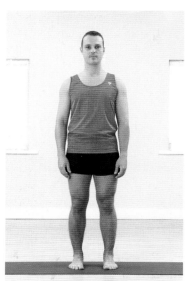

1 Mountain Pose (4 breaths)

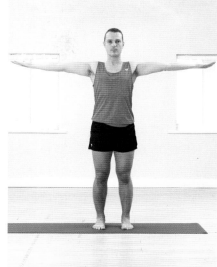

2 Complete Breath (x1)

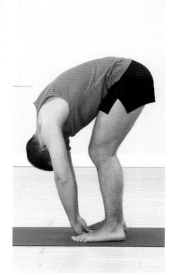

3 Refresher Breath (x1)

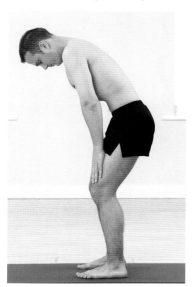

4 Abdominal Lift (x1)

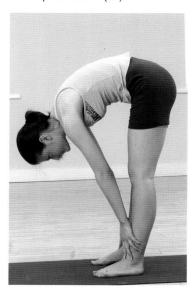

5 Standing Forward Bend 1 (x1)

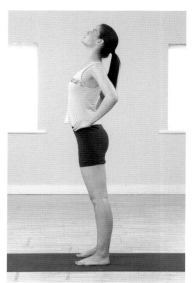

6 Standing Backward Bend (x1)

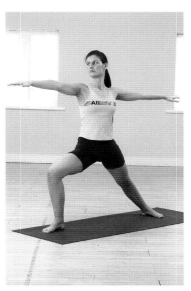

7 Warrior, pose 1 (x1)

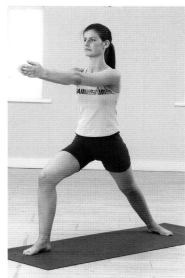

8 Warrior, pose 2 (x1)

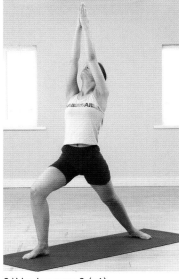

9 Warrior, pose 3 (x1)

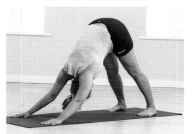

10 Downward Dog (x1)

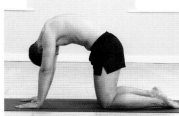

12 Cat (x1)

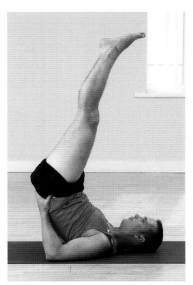

14 Half Shoulder Stand (x1)

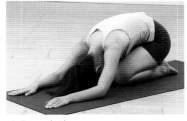

11 Swan (x1)

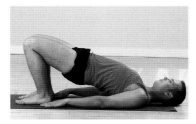

13 Modified Back Bend (x3)

sequence 7 (continued)

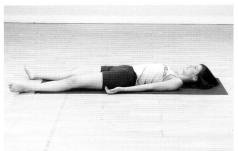

15 Relaxed pose (4 breaths)

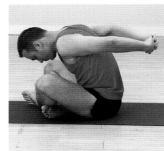

16 Lotus Forward Bend (x1)

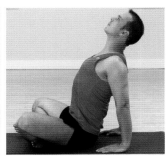

17 Lotus Backward Bend (1 breath)

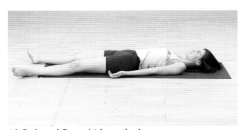

18 Relaxed Pose (4 breaths)

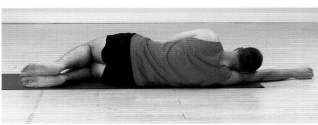

19 Curl Up (x1)

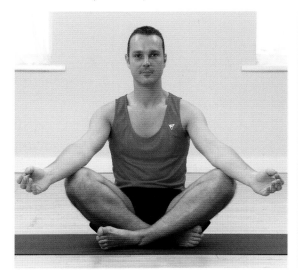

20 Sit Up (x1)

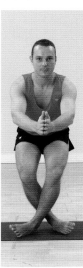

21 Stand Up (x1)

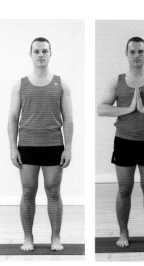

22 Mountain Pose (4 breaths)
23 Closing Breath

As you practice and make progress you will feel your flexibility increasing. Now is the time to include poses 1 and 2 in the Standing and Seated Forward Bends. For example in Sequence 1, follow Standing Forward Bend 1 with 2 and 3 when you feel you are able.

Remember it's not about touching your toes at all costs. It's about lengthening and stretching, and responding to the needs of the moment. You may find some days you feel as supple as a piece of elastic, and other days, as stiff as a board. So choose your sequence with sensitivity to your needs and abilities.

It is normal procedure in yoga to refrain from any practice for the first three days of menstruation. Instead, practice relaxation, concentration, and meditation. Also, never forget when you are menstruating that your hips should never be higher than your heart. So no Modified Back Bend or Half Shoulder Stand (inverted poses).

Once you are familiar with the names, breathing, and techniques of the poses, you can create your own sequence. Always complement a Forward Bend with its contrapose a Backward Bend, so that the spine arches in opposite directions. For example, the Fish is a contrapose to the Coil. If you practice to the right. The contrapose is to the left.

All the postures include instructions on how to arrive at the pose, hold the pose, and leave the pose. With the exception of Downward Dog, which is entered from Warrior 1 and exits through the Swan.

In time, you will be able to practice the sequence which includes all the postures in this book. It will take you approximately one hour. If you include deep relaxation, concentration and meditation allow yourself one and a half hours.

Sensitivity, grace, ease, a calm mind, and a quiet breath are yoga's gifts that you can practice anywhere any time. The moment you become aware of your breathing rhythm, you are practicing yoga. So do not beat yourself up on the days you do not feel like practicing the postures. Listen to your breathing and enjoy your life to the best of your abilities. We are here to have fun and live fulfilling, happy lives.

Developing the Postures

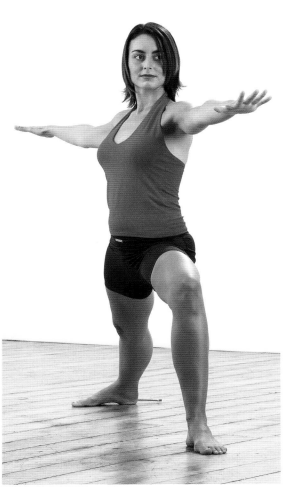

In order to develop the postures and yoga skills we have to practice and persevere, even when we think it's not worth it and we just cannot be bothered. It is at exactly these times, if we can muster our intent, get focused, and listen to our breathing, that we will make our greatest progress. Our Forward Bend might not be perfect, but you are still practicing. Heaven is right where you are standing, and that is the place to train. Constant practice and perseverance are the greatest skills we can develop. They are the tools that enable us to enjoy our life.

The discipline required to practice on a regular basis comes from focus and concentration and the firm determination to do something about your life. Yoga is as much about stretching the perimeters of your mind as it is about stretching your spine.

We should always breathe in through the nostrils and out through the nostrils (unless you are practicing a specific technique or you are blocked up with a cold). This may be difficult at first but again, persevere.

The first sign of progress is a quiet mind. This is demonstrated in the softness of the face, the rhythm of the breath, and alignment of the spine. It is the constant repetition of the postures which increases flexibility and this has a corresponding stretching effect on the mind.

When our breath is calm, our mind is calm. In order to develop and reap the benefits of our yoga practice, we must start with the right attitude.

We should be relaxed and looking forward to our practice. It is easy to think we are relaxed, but often we are holding stress and tensions we are unaware of.

So, you may find it beneficial to begin with a method specifically designed to rid you of these tensions. In this exercise we will consciously tense, then relax the muscles in order to learn to recognize the difference between tension and relaxation.

You may practice the Method of Relaxation either before or after your practice. You may like to practice this method alone, when you need to catch up with yourself, take time out, de-stress, refresh, and revitalize. This is a wonderful technique for calming the mind and leaves us feeling harmonious, relaxed, and at peace with ourselves and the world. The relaxed pose also prepares you for concentration and meditation.

The Deep Relaxation Method

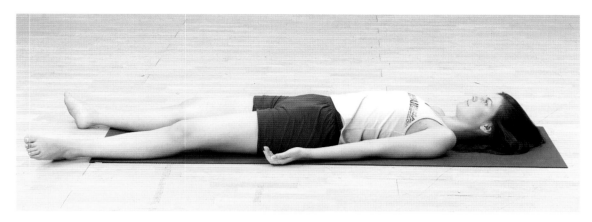

We will tense each part of the body in turn and then relax each part.

1 Lie, supine on the floor, in Relaxed Pose; legs and feet apart, feet wider than the hips. Move your arms away from your sides with the back of your head to the floor, eyes directly to the sky. Make yourself as comfortable as you can.

2 Breathe comfortably.

3 Tense each part of the body in turn and then relax each part, starting with your hands.

The hands:

4 Make your hands into tightly-clenched fists, clench them tight, tighter, feel the tension in your hands and arms; then, let your hands relax. The back of your hands are on the floor. Your fingers are lightly curled.

The arms:

5 Now, stretch out your fingers away from you. Straighten your arms, feel the tension in your hands, arms, shoulders, and let them relax. The back of your arms and hands are on the floor. Your fingers are lightly curled.

6 Breathe comfortably.

The upper arms:

7 Bend your arms at your elbows and try to press your wrists to your shoulders. Feel the tension in your shoulders and upper spine and let your arms drop

back down to the floor. Relax your arms completely. The back of your hands are on the floor.

8 Let any tensions ease away from the muscles in your arms, noticing the difference between tension and relaxation. Carry on the feeling of letting go. Your arms are beginning to feel heavier and heavier as they sink into the floor and relax more and more.

The shoulders:

9 Shrug your shoulders up toward your neck. Let your shoulders drop right down. Feel the difference, as tension eases away from you, enjoy the feeling of letting go.

10 With the back of your head to the floor, eyes to the ceiling, feel yourself sinking into the floor.

The face:

11 Raise your eyebrows as high as you can, really wrinkling your forehead. Hold and relax. Let your eyebrows drop. Imagine the skin across your forehead and scalp becoming smoother and smoother as you relax and let go.

12 Now frown as hard as you can, bringing the eyebrows together and wrinkling your forehead. Hold, relax your forehead and let go. Allow the brow to become smooth and unwrinkled.

The eyes:

13 Close your eyes and clench them tightly shut. Squeeze them tightly together. Feel the tension and relax.

Relax the eyelids so they are just touching the lower lashes, with no tension and no effort.

The jaw:

14 Gently press the top and bottom teeth together. Hold for one full breath and relax. Let your lower jaw drop.

15 Breathe comfortably.

Throat and tongue:

16 Press the tip of your tongue firmly to the roof of your mouth behind the top teeth. Hold and relax. Let your tongue drop.

The lips:

17 Press your lips together as tight as you can. Then relax—your lips rest just lightly apart. No tensions, no effort in your face.

The chest:

18 Take a breath in and out.

19 Breathe in, hold your breath.

20 Breathe in a little more, hold your breath.

21 Breathe out through your mouth with a big sigh.

22 Breathe comfortably and smoothly, not too deep.

The stomach:

23 Breathe in and out.

24 Draw your navel toward your spine.

25 Draw your stomach inward and upward.

26 Relax your stomach, let go, and feel the tension ease away. Breathe in and out.

27 Stretch your toes away from you. Feel the tension in your thighs, knees, calves, ankles, feet, and toes (don't overdo it—you don't want to cause a cramp in your legs or toes).

28 Let your legs and feet relax. Legs and feet apart. Breathe easy/normally.

Each time you breathe out, feel yourself sinking deeper and deeper into the floor. Each time you breathe out, feel yourself relax more and more. If any tension has crept back in, tell that part to relax and let go.

Keep your fingers and hands relaxed. Keep your arms and shoulders relaxed and at ease. Keep all the muscles in your face and head completely relaxed, completely at ease.

Feel your chest sinking toward the floor. Feel your stomach relax, thighs, calves, ankles, feet, and toes are all completely relaxed. Listen to your breathing. Become aware how much deeper, smoother, and calmer your breathing has become.

When you feel ready, roll yourself into a seated pose and sit in a comfortable position.

The Method of Concentration

When the mind and body are relaxed and unified with the rhythm of your breath, you can focus and concentrate.

He who devotes himself to the path of concentration, aims the arrow of awareness and releases it upon the true center within. For when all the scattered impressions of thought and feelings are drawn together into the unity of yoga, they become a force to be reckoned with. If a thousand men fight and squabble with each other, the result is a vast waste of energy, but if they all pull together resolutely for a common cause, their combined power can move mountains. This is the secret of yoga and anything the student can do to bring all the scattered forces within his domain together, in obedience to his will, is a move towards unity.

John Gent

Concentration is pinpointing the mind on an object and that which is immediately associated with it; whereas meditation is pinpointing the mind on the very essence of an object by excluding all other thoughts. Concentration is an aid to meditation in that it harnesses and preserves our energies which would otherwise be wasted in involvement with the body image. When we practice Yoga, we use our powers of concentration in an effort to achieve a meditative state of being. As the mind is apt to wander, and a multitude of worldly thoughts invade our being, we concentrate on a particular thing or aspect. This will focus our attention, ridding us of negative thoughts and frustrations, and create a feeling of clarity in the mind.

This can be achieved by concentration on the breath, on enunciation of a sound (mantra) such as "om." Gaze at an object, such as a flower, shell, or the flame of a candle. You can concentrate on a particular part of the body, directing healing light to that part to help alleviate pain and tension. You can concentrate on anything that keeps other thoughts out of your mind, such as the sound of the rain, the sound of the wind, the song of a bird. The idea of these aids is that after time, you will arrive at, and remain in, a peaceful and tranquil state of being.

1 Sit in a comfortable position, eyes forward, and spine erect.
2 Imagine a golden thread, running from the base of the spine, up the spine, out the top of your head, and drawing your spine toward heaven—supporting and lengthening your spine.
3 Breathe comfortably.
4 Listen to your breathing. Become aware of the rise of your chest as you breathe in and the fall of your chest as you breathe out.
5 Notice the quality of your breath. Is it deep, smooth, and rhythmic?
6 Be aware of the movement of your lungs. Breathing in, expanding. Breathing out, contracting. Filling and emptying. Union. Rhythm. Peace.
7 Stay seated, comfortable, ready for meditation.

The practice of concentration brings peace of mind, strengthens our resolve, and increases our powers of observation. Concentration is the "asana" of the mind. It is an exercise whereby we are aware of our focus of attention. In this case, it is the breath and also its associated qualities, such as sound, quality, and rhythm. By identifying with an object, we become one with it. That is why I like my concentration to be on my breath, because I can practice anywhere, any time, with no aids.

The Method of Meditation

The aim of meditation is to achieve peace of mind and a quiet spirit. The objective is to rid yourself of all verbal, physical, and mental violence.

The result is a preservation of your energies (prana or life force) which is otherwise wasted in unnecessary involvement with the body image. We attain self-control and self harmony.

Meditation exercise is a way of life for millions of people in India, Tibet, Korea, China, Japan, and throughout the Eastern world. The meditative practices of t'ai chi ch'uan are practiced on a daily basis in parks and village squares, where most of the population will join in, regardless of age. They practice for the health of body and mind, and peace of spirit. Through the perfection of action, we learn self-control, which is self harmony, which allows us to live in harmony with other people. In the West we often misunderstand the practice of meditation, thinking we must cut ourselves off from the world and sit in a cross-legged position.

Meditation, in which the senses are brought under control, the perfection of self-harmony, is the essence of karma yoga. Karma yoga is sacred work. In this way, meditation is finding peace in everything you do. As long as you find yourself doing a particular thing, you might as well enjoy it. Offer your work as a sacrifice to the infinite (or universe). Do not think about what you could be doing, be aware of what you *are* doing and find peace in it.

Meditation is the union of the finite with the infinite, and the harmony created from this joining and merging of opposites.

The reconciliation of the finite with the infinite, the union between matter and life force (prana) are other ways of describing the union, the cosmic intercourse (nada) between father (shiva) and mother (shakti).

"Just as the vibrations of intercourse produces seminal fluid, which unites with the female egg to create a new being, so cosmic nada enlivens the cosmic egg, to produce a viable living universe." Hathapradipika.

Meditation is creative. When psychic energies are withdrawn from the peripheral systems and concentrated in the central areas of the brain, an altered state of consciousness is created.

We experience sat, vit, and ananda—being, consciousness, and joy.

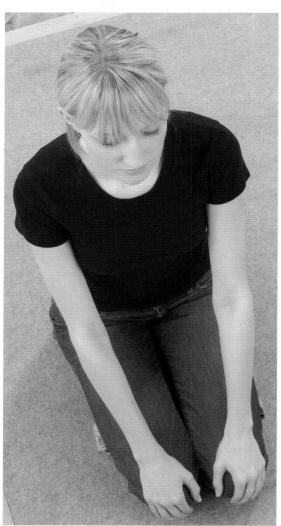

Seated Meditation

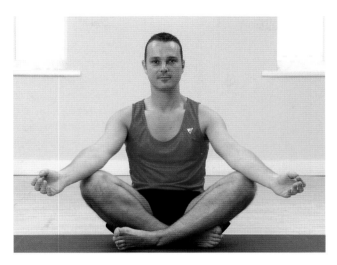

1 Sit with your spine erect.

2 With your thumb and first fingers touching, rest the backs of your hands on your thighs or knees. Keep your breathing deep and rhythmic.

3 Listen to your breathing and close your eyes. Take your attention to ajna chakra, your third eye, situated in the middle of your forehead, between the eyebrows.

4 Imagine this area suffused with white light. It is as if you are looking inward. Inside yourself.

5 Become one with this white light. Meditate on light. You are light. Whole, safe, and secure. You are loved.

6 Stay like this for a minimum of five minutes.

7 When you are ready, breathe more deeply and swallow one or two times.

8 As you slowly come out of meditation, that is when your mind starts wandering again, keep that feeling of love and peace within you, let love and peace be your mantra for the day.

9 Begin to breathe more deeply.

10 Briskly rub your hands together and place them over your eyes.

11 Open your fingers and open your eyes. Let the light shine through.

12 Practice hair tugs and stroke your face.

13 When you are ready, stand up and have a good stretch.

Remember, after meditation, before you rejoin the world of activity, practice the Closing Breath three times, so light, love, and energy stay within you, stored, preserved, for as and when we need it. Meditation can help us develop incredible physical and mental stamina.

As you practice more and more often, appreciating the wonderful way meditation can light up your life, you will find the ability to sit quietly, concentrate, and meditate easier and easier. You will sit in meditation for longer periods of time, not because you are forcing yourself to do so, but because it is the most natural thing to do.

Beyond the junkshop of the mind there lies a curtained, inner room.

Here, the hurt soul can reach again and touch a bloom,

Unbruised by grasping hands outside.

Take off your shoes,

Bring nothing in

Fold your costume harlequin,

The masquerading self has died.

The Buddha

157

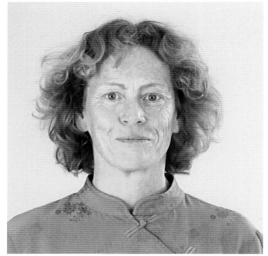

are the most rewarding. The effort put in and the delight and satisfaction of these students as they respond to challenges and new ways of thinking puts most of us to shame. What I love about yoga is that it is a great equalizer between people, as there is always something you can excel at. In fact, it is often those who are less able, who really gain the benefits of yoga, because they make such quantum leaps.

So don't worry about how you look in your yoga gear, how stiff and unfit you are, or how unsociable you feel. Get moving onto your yoga mat or get off to your class and get on with it.

Don't let indecision and uncertainty stand in your way. I practice yoga every morning for twenty minutes and in the evening before bed, another five minutes of slow, easy stretching, like Forward Bends to ease out any tensions. Often I will increase the amount of time I practice, for example I may go to a weekend workshop myself, or go to daily Astanga classes when I am teaching at centers around the world. Mostly I practice just because I want to, because it makes me feel so good.

I hope this book inspires you to learn about, practice, and understand the art of yoga. This is the first step on your journey to realization and happiness.

The path I chose

I have been practicing yoga since I was 14 years old. My mom went to yoga classes and it was she who got me started on the yogic path. I have been practicing ever since. I believe in yoga. I know first hand of its wonderful benefits. I find that yoga is a fantastic complement to all other activities, such as running, tennis, swimming, martial arts, public speaking, sitting quietly, or writing a book. You name it, the practice of yoga will enhance your life.

There has been a phenomenal growth in interest in yoga in the past five years. More and more people are practicing just as more and more people are teaching. There are yoga classes in all the gyms and health clubs. Unfortunately, this has led to many aerobic and dance instructors jumping on the bandwagon and setting up classes, when they have no qualifications or experience to teach such a specialized, traditional art. It is paramount to find a qualified instructor.

Teaching yoga, like the practice itself, is a joy. I often teach at weekends where there can be up to 150 people in each class. All those people breathing in unison and all focused on love and light is fantastic.

Participating in a yoga class is a lovely experience, and is a chance to meet the like-minded and make new friends. For the physically or mentally challenged, the ill of health and the elderly, I must admit, these classes

Bibliography

The Hathapradipika, Kevin and Venika Kingsland
Kung Fu Meditations, Ellen Li Hua
The Bhagavad Gita, translated by Juan Mascaro
Yoga, John Gent
The Art of Peace, Morihei Ueshiba
The Seeker's Guide to Nutrition, Tony Thornley

I would like to dedicate this book to my mum and dad and say thanks to Gayle Tucker, Gordon, Gay, Lottie, Kevin, and my sister Annie, for their support and encouragement.

Index

index continued

Acknowledgments

All images © Chrysalis Image Library / Mike Prior except for the following.

© Chrysalis Image Library / Eddie MacDonald 16, 21, 23, 37, 127, 152, 156. / Kuo kang Chen 6, 8.

© CORBIS: © Jutta Klee/CORBIS 7. / © Jim Craigmyle/CORBIS 10. / © Pete Saloutos/CORBIS 11. / © LWA-Dann Tardif/CORBIS 12, 19.

Chrysalis Books Group Plc is committed to respecting the intellectual property rights of others. We have therefore taken all reasonable efforts to ensure that the reproduction of all content on these pages is done with the full consent of copyright owners. If you are aware of any unintentional omissions please contact the company directly so that any necessary corrections may be made for future editions.